BURNS

A PRACTICAL APPROACH TO IMMEDIATE TREATMENT AND LONG-TERM CARE

ROB SHERIDAN MD

Burn Surgery Service, Boston Shriners Hospital for Children
Division of Burns, Massachusetts General Hospital
Department of Surgery, Harvard Medical School
Boston, Massachusetts, USA

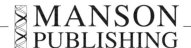

DEDICATION

'The family is a haven in a heartless world.'
Christopher Lasch 1932–1994, historian, philosopher, writer

'You don't choose your family. They are God's gift to you, as you are to them.'
Desmond Tutu (1931–present), South African cleric and social activist,
winner of the Nobel Peace Prize

To Martha, Kevin, Danny, and Anna Mae

Author proceeds from sales of this book will be donated directly to Shriners Hospitals for Children.

Note: Every effort has been made to eliminate inaccuracies but readers are advised to confirm recommended doses in the drug data sheets before prescribing regimens. Reader's comments, suggestions and a note of any errors will be appreciated.

The advice and information given in this book are believed to be true and accurate at the time of going to press, but neither the author nor the publisher can accept any legal responsibility or liability for any errors or omissions that have been made.

A CIP catalogue record for this book is available from the British Library.

For full details of all Manson Publishing Ltd titles please write to:
Manson Publishing Ltd, 73 Corringham Road, London NW11 7DL, UK.
Tel: +44(0)20 8905 5150
Fax: +44(0)20 8201 9233
Website: www.mansonpublishing.com

Commissioning editor: Jill Northcott
Project manager: Paul Bennett
Copy-editor: Ruth Maxwell
Design and layout: Cathy Martin
Colour reproduction: Tenon & Polert Colour Scanning Ltd, Hong Kong
Printed by: Grafos S.A., Barcelona

Contents

PREFACE

'The medical professionals who treat burns are a multidisciplinary team of dedicated healers doing punishing work for little in the way of glory or riches.'
Barbara Ravage in *Burn Unit*.

'We should always let our judgments and recommendations be guided by the fact that we operate on patients, not on diseases.'
Stanley O. Hoerr, former Chief of Surgery, Cleveland Clinic.

Burns are very common injuries. Virtually every health care provider will be called upon to help burn patients through some part of the acute or recovery phases of their injuries. Pediatric and adult medical specialists, emergency medicine practitioners, general and plastic and pediatric surgeons, visiting and in-patient nurses, occupational and physical therapists, physiatrists and psychiatrists, all will interface with burn patients. It is very helpful to understand what they have been through and where they are going. However, the particular audience for this book is the surgeons and burn team members who will be providing overall direction and procedural care to burned individuals. This monograph focuses on practical fundamentals of clinical burn care. When such principles can be consistently applied, most of our patients do very well. Further, a consistent program of practical care forms a stable foundation upon which new innovations are more likely to succeed.

Rob Sheridan MD

ACKNOWLEDGEMENTS

'The patients in the wards presented the usual clinical picture of large exposed burn wounds covered by broken-down eschars, with infected granulating areas on anemic, exhausted and frightened individuals.'
Dr. Zora Janzekovic, burn surgeon and early excision pioneer, on her experience caring for burn patients in the 1950s and 1960s.

'Shun no science, scorn no book, nor cling fanatically to a single creed.'
The Brothers of Purity, 10th century Shiite Muslims.

Over the past 20 years, I have had the privilege to have been a member of two great burn care organizations, the United States Army's Institute of Surgical Research and the Harvard burn program at the Boston Shriners Hospital for Children, Massachusetts General Hospital, and Brigham and Women's Hospital. Even in my short career, I have witnessed substantial improvement in many areas of burn care and have seen many of these translate into enhanced outcomes for our patients. I am indebted to my colleagues for their friendship. I am indebted to my patients and their families for their lessons. Most of all, I am indebted to my family for their love and support.

Rob Sheridan MD

CHAPTER 1

BACKGROUND

'If you can't describe what you are doing as a process, you don't know what you are doing.'

W. Edwards Deming (1900–1993),
industrial process and quality control pioneer.

'It's amazing how much you can accomplish if you don't care who gets the credit.'

Harry S. Truman (1884–1972),
American President.

Few fields have changed more in the past few decades than burns. Through the hard work of those who have gone before, a depressing lonely field, littered with routine tragedies, has become an exciting multi-disciplinary calling, saving lives and restoring function. But these good outcomes only come if providers are skilled in the basics. No expensive new product can replace a solid understanding of the fundamentals of burn care, learned at a high price by providers and patients who have gone before. The purpose of this monograph is to review those fundamentals, so burn care providers can have a platform upon which to build the enhanced outcomes of the future.

RECENT HISTORY

Without intervention, patients with serious burns die for three primary reasons. Burn shock in the first day, respiratory failure in the following 3–5 days, and burn wound sepsis in subsequent weeks. Over the past 60 years, thoughtful clinicians have identified and addressed each of these issues, changing the natural history of the injury (**1, 2**).

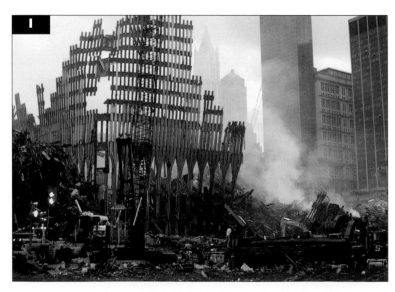

1 Throughout history, those faced with fire disasters have provided us with valuable lessons in how best to manage these situations and patients. Unfortunately, disastrous fires continue to occur. Burn care providers should continuously be prepared to assist. In the aftermath of the World Trade Center incident in 2001, the concept of secondary triage of burn patients evolved.

Burn shock was clearly described by those caring for mass burn casualties in fires such as the Rialto Concert Hall and Cocoanut Grove fires in the 1930s and 1940s (see Textbox: Disasters). Based on these experiences, weight and burn size-based resuscitation formulas were developed and then refined in the 1950s and 1960s. Based on this work, burn shock has become a relatively infrequent cause of death in those who arrive at a site of definitive care within 24 hours of injury.

It was during this same era, particularly after the Cocoanut Grove fire, that respiratory failure following inhalation of toxic fumes was appreciated as a clinical entity. The subsequent development of mechanical ventilation and its application to burn victims has reduced respiratory failure as a cause of death, although this problem still plagues the field. The reduction in wound sepsis as an early cause of burn-related death is a central accomplishment in burn care. This work was pioneered in Eastern Europe in the 1960s and 1970s, where small deep burns were excised and grafted upon recognition, rather than waiting until burns sloughed to granulating fat. This work was extended to patients with large burns in the United States and elsewhere in subsequent decades, this exercise requiring extensive blood bank and intensive care unit support. Early recognition and excision of deep burns remains a central concept that profoundly modifies the natural history of burns.

DISASTERS

Victims of burn disasters have not suffered and died completely in vain. Burn care providers faced with horrors such as the Triangle Shirtwaist Factory Fire, Rialto Concert Hall Fire, Hartford Circus Fire, Cocoanut Grove Fire, Station Nightclub Fire, and incendiary warfare since World War One have eked painful lessons from these and other tragedies. This knowledge has led to safer buildings, better resuscitation formulas, improved pain control, increasingly prompt wound closure, improved recovery skills, more sophisticated patient flow, and better preparation for the next disaster.

2 The burn unit skill set is valuable in managing the soft tissue injuries which dominate in survivors of natural disasters and terrorist incidents. Large numbers of complex soft tissue injuries, such as pictured here from the 2010 Haiti earthquake, occur in nonburn disasters. The burn unit skill set is very important in these scenarios.

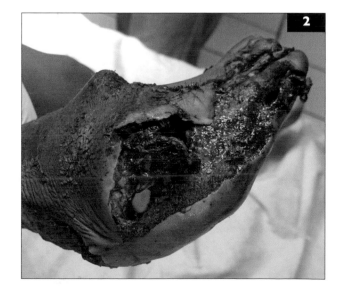

EPIDEMIOLOGY

Burns are common injuries. It is estimated that for about 3.5 million people there should be one burn unit. In the United States each year, approximately 2 million people are injured, 80,000 are hospitalized, and 6,500 die from burns. The mechanisms vary with age and socioeconomic status. Approximately 70% of pediatric burns are caused by hot liquid, whereas flame injuries more often cause burns in working aged adults. The very young and the very old are at increased risk for burns, commonly in kitchen or bathing accidents. Up to 20% of injuries in young children involve abuse or neglect. All suspicious injuries should be reported to state authorities.

ORGANIZATION OF BURN CARE

Complex surgical problems are most cost effectively managed in high volume programs. This 'volume-outcome effect' is supported by a growing body of evidence in burn care. Burn care requires personnel and equipment that are not cost effectively maintained in low volume programs. In North America, these issues have led to the formation of the burn center verification program, a combined effort of the American Burn Association and American College of Surgeons. Patients with serious burns are increasingly sent to regional programs for care. The growing emphasis is on comprehensive care for all aspects of the burn condition in one multidisciplinary program. The American Burn Association has developed a set of criteria suggesting which patients should be referred to regional burn centers (*Table 1*). Care of patients with large complex burn injuries can be subdivided into four general phases, each with specific objectives. This process helps to define short-term goals during long processes of care (*Table 2*).

LONG-TERM OUTCOMES

Survival of patients with large burns has improved dramatically over recent decades. These changes have been so rapid, that long-term outcome quality is poorly understood. One report of a large number of massively burned survivors with 15 years of follow-up demonstrated that most had a very high quality of survival when they participated in a comprehensive long-term aftercare program. It is clearly possible for burn survivors to lead happy and productive lives. However, it appears that achieving such outcomes for those surviving very serious burns requires a coordinated multidisciplinary effort by a team of burn surgeons, physical and occupational therapists, nurses, anesthesiologists, social workers, recreational therapists, and mental health professionals who work well together as a team. The need for such teams has led to the concentration of seriously burned patients in large regional centers, which facilitates maintenance of needed expertise. This 'holistic' approach to burn care, in which not just survival but long-term quality survival is the care team's goal, has an important impact on outcome quality. New outcome study tools have demonstrated the importance of the environment of recovery, including family dynamics (Textbox: Environment of recovery).

ENVIRONMENT OF RECOVERY

Recovery from a serious burn only just begins with wound closure, survival, and physical recovery. Increasingly sophisticated long-term outcome studies have demonstrated the crucial role of emotional recovery. The impact of a supportive environment can make the difference between chronic emotional suffering and isolation, and productive contentment and full reintegration for burn survivors. Organizations such as the Phoenix Society for Burn Survivors can help providers and patients access the resources needed to enjoy full physical and emotional recovery (see page 118, Textbox: The Guinea Pig Club).

Table 1 American Burn Association Burn Center transfer criteria*

- Second- and third-degree burns greater than 10% total body surface area (TBSA) in patients under 10 or over 50 years of age
- Second- and third-degree burns greater than 20% TBSA in other age groups
- Second- and third-degree burns that involve the face, hands, feet, genitalia, perineum, and major joints
- Third-degree burns greater than 5% TBSA in any age group
- Electrical burns including lightning injury
- Chemical burns
- Inhalation injury
- Burn injury in patients with pre-existing medical disorders that could complicate management, prolong recovery, or affect mortality
- Any patients with burns and concomitant trauma (such as fractures) in which the burn injury poses the greatest risk of morbidity or mortality. In such cases, if the trauma poses the greater immediate risk, the patient may be treated initially in a trauma center until stable before being transferred to a burn center. Physician judgment will be necessary in such situations and should be in concert with the regional medical control plan and triage protocols
- Hospitals without qualified personnel or equipment for the care of children should transfer children with burns to a burn center with these capabilities
- Burn injury in patients who will require special social/emotional and/or long-term rehabilitative support, including cases involving suspected child abuse, substance abuse

*The UK and Europe generally follow the Advanced Trauma Life Support (ATLS) guidelines (see page 19). Referral criteria are more or less identical to the above

Table 2 Phases of burn care

In-patient care of larger burns has four general phases. The duration and intensity of each phase will vary with wound extent and complexity. Short-term objectives of each phase are listed here:

Initial evaluation and resuscitation (0–72 hr):
- Clearly identify all injuries
- Perform an accurate individualized fluid resuscitation
- Ensure effective decompression of extremities and torso

Initial excision and biologic closure (days 1–7):
- Accurately identify all wounds requiring surgery
- Excise the bulk of all full-thickness wounds
- Effect definitive or temporary biologic closure of wounds created by excision

Definitive wound closure (weeks 1–6):
- Replace temporary wound membranes with permanent coverage
- Close physiologically small, but functionally critical areas (e.g. hands and face)
- Separate patient from intensive care support

Rehabilitation and reconstruction (day 1–year 2):
- Initiate early ranging, splinting and antideformity positioning
- Progress to active strength and endurance training
- Initiate scar management program
- Foster reintegration with family and community

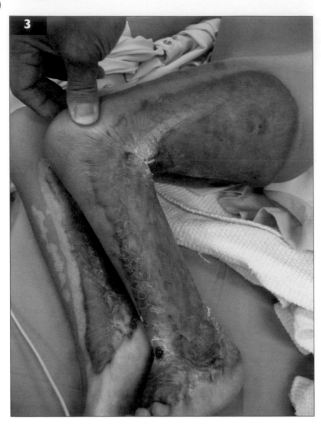

3 Caring for burn patients in resource-limited settings is very difficult; the natural history of the injuries dominates clinical outcomes.

AUSTERE ALTERNATIVES

This book is written from the perspective of a burn program where resources are usually abundant. Most practitioners of burn care are not so fortunate and are faced daily with difficult resource allocation decisions. Burns must often be left to heal by a slow and painful process of contraction and epithelialization. All too often, crippling deformity can result. Surgeons working in these settings are faced with very limited access to the operating room to close acute wounds and reconstruct established deformities. Some will be able to work with charitable organizations to help provide these needed resources. Examples in Central America include the Ruth Paz Foundation in Honduras and the ARPOQUEN Foundation in Nicaragua. Circumstances cause them to become skilled at clinical compromise.

While a young Army general surgeon stationed in Central America in the 1980s I had some exposure to these realities. Subsequent opportunities to operate and visit general surgery and burn programs in Central America and Indonesia have given me some limited experiences in this regard. I have learned that any differences in outcomes between patients managed in the developing world and those managed in our resource-rich setting are certainly not based on differences in surgical talent. To address some of these important realities with the reader, the editor has suggested that an 'Austere Alternatives' section be added to each chapter. In these paragraphs, with great humility and respect, I have tried to offer suggestions to those who are resource challenged. I would be grateful for any feedback to make this section more useful in a subsequent edition of this monograph. Those caring for burn patients in the developing world are the real heroes of our specialty (**3**).

CHAPTER 2

PHYSIOLOGY OF BURNS

'There resulted from this local injury a great
constitutional disturbance.'
> Surgeon Daniel Drake MD (1785–1852),
> describing his own burn injury in 1830.
> (See Textbox: Daniel Drake's burn.)

'Fortune favors the prepared mind.'
> Louis Pasteur (1822–95),
> French chemist and microbiologist.

Most of us do not adequately appreciate our skin, subjecting this miraculous and precious membrane to disdain and abuse. Our epidermal layer provides a vapor and bacterial barrier, while our dermis provides the skin's flexibility and strength. The durable bonding between these layers is crucial, as demonstrated by those disease processes in which the bond is temporarily or permanently lost, such as toxic epidermal necrolysis and epidermolysis bullosa.

Dermal appendages prevent desiccation of the skin by producing oils and the reactive dermal microvasculature facilitates heat dissipation and conservation. All these essential functions are deranged when substantial areas of the skin are burned. Further, large burns drive poorly understood systemic inflammatory and catabolic processes that in themselves can be quite destructive.

LOCAL RESPONSE TO BURN INJURY

At the sites of burn, there are both immediate and progressive injuries. Immediate changes are primarily coagulation of involved tissues. In the following hours, uncoagulated tissues on the periphery are subject to a variable degree of microvascular thrombosis and ischemia, deepening and extending the injury to some degree. Despite research with

DANIEL DRAKE'S BURN

Dr. Daniel Drake was raised in a one-room cabin in the Kentucky wilderness of post-Revolutionary War America. A bright child, he was influenced by a local doctor to study medicine at the University of Pennsylvania. He became a widely recognized surgeon, traveling, teaching, and operating throughout the mid-West. He was a prolific writer on surgical topics. In his later years he wrote a fascinating series of letters to his children describing his pioneer life which was republished as recently as 1999. On September 18th 1828, he attempted to extinguish the burning mosquito netting of his sister-in-law, who did not survive the episode. His heroic attempt caused severe burns to his hands. He wrote a riveting commentary describing his injury and its sequela. It is one of the earliest descriptions of the pain and profound systemic disturbance caused by a serious burn.

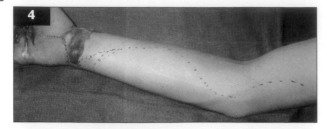

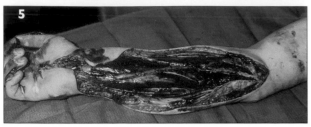

4, 5 Avoidance of burn shock, hypothermia, and reduced inflow from increased soft tissue pressures will prevent exacerbation of secondary injury. This extremity was effectively decompressed by fasciotomy 3 hr after high-voltage injury. There is a very limited amount of muscle damage at this point (dark muscle). However, extensive amounts of muscle are very edematous. Had fasciotomy not been performed, far worse secondary injury would have resulted from intracompartmental hypertension and ischemia.

CUTHBERSTON'S INJURY PHASES

In the early 1940s, while studying urinary excretion of minerals in fracture patients, Scottish nutritional scientist David Cuthbertson demonstrated the catabolic response to injury. Although this response had been clinically noted as early as the 18th century by Sir John Hunter, Cuthbertson was the first to clearly document 'ebb' and 'flow' phases of injury. His ebb phase, a hypodynamic period more notable in poorly resuscitated patients, is predictably followed in surviving patients by a flow phase, characterized by a hyperdynamic circulation and muscle catabolism. Cuthbertson developed a crest for his Institute of Nutritional Study at the University of Aberdeen that featured the phrase, 'Understand and Nourish'. These goals of injury care apply to this day. Cuthbertson was later knighted for his work.

antioxidants and wound cooling, no intervention is known to ameliorate reliably this secondary local ischemia. Avoidance of burn shock, hypothermia, and reduced inflow from increased soft tissue pressures will prevent exacerbation of secondary injury (**4, 5**).

As bacteria multiply in the avascular tissue over the days following injury, proteases liquefy the eschar which then separates, leaving a bed of granulation tissue or healing burn depending on the depth of the original injury. In healthy patients with small (<20% of the body surface) burns, this septic process is usually tolerated. When injuries are larger, systemic inflammation and infection result, explaining the rare survival of patients with burns in excess of 40% of the body surface managed without early wound excision and closure.

SYSTEMIC RESPONSE TO BURN INJURY

The systemic response to injury is increasingly disruptive as burns affect more than about 20% of the body surface. Barrier function is lost, with associated fluid and electrolyte depletion and decreased resistance to infection. Vasoactive mediators are released from the injured tissues with diffuse interstitial edema and organ dysfunction. Bacteria proliferate within avascular eschar with resulting systemic inflammation and infection.

Patients with large burns demonstrate an initial decrease in cardiac output and metabolic rate (the 'ebb phase'). In the days following injury those who have been successfully resuscitated develop a stereotypical hypermetabolic response (the 'flow phase'), with near doubling of cardiac output and resting energy expenditure. Enhanced gluconeogenesis, insulin resistance, and increased protein catabolism are seen and have major implications for the care of burn patients. This physiology is not well understood but is felt to involve changes in hypothalamic function with coincident increases in glucagon, cortisol, and catecholamine secretion, deficient gastrointestinal barrier function with translocation of bacteria and their byproducts, bacterial contamination of the burn wound with systemic release of their products, and

6 Without nutritional intervention, the hypermetabolic response will predictably lead to inanition in initial survivors of serious burns. The cachectic state, as illustrated here, will compromise chances of survival. Ongoing nutritional support is a cornerstone of successful burn care.

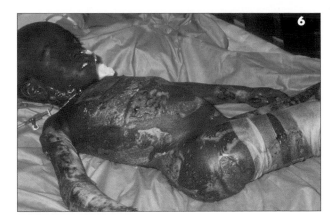

enhanced heat loss via transeschar evaporation. The cornerstone of management of this hypermetabolic response is adequate nutritional support. Modification of the hypermetabolic response has been hindered by our poor understanding of the basic biology. Beta-adrenergic blockade, nonsteroidal anti-inflammatory drugs (NSAIDs), growth hormone, anabolic steroids, and insulin-like growth factor-1 are under active investigation. Currently available data are not adequate to support the routine use of therapies designed to modify the hypermetabolic response. Support of the response through nutrition remains the clinical imperative (**6**).

PEDIATRIC CONSIDERATIONS

Young children bring unique physiologic issues to the burn unit (*Table 3*). Injury mechanisms are weighted toward scalding, particularly in younger children. The possibility of abuse must always be considered, and if conditions are suspicious, children should be admitted for further evaluation and state authorities notified.

The smaller pediatric upper airway is more rapidly occluded by progressive edema. Stridor and retractions should trigger immediate evaluation and possible intubation. The trachea of the young child is short, making mainstem intubation common. Bronchospasm is much more frequently an issue in young children after inhalation injury, and should be addressed to avoid respiratory fatigue and dynamic hyperinflation. Children have a thinner skin than adults. Burns are relatively deeper and donor sites more unforgiving of a deep pass with a dermatome.

Table 3 Pediatric considerations
- The smaller pediatric upper airway is more readily occluded by edema
- Injury mechanisms more commonly involve abuse or neglect
- The short trachea of the young child makes mainstem intubation common
- Bronchospasm is more commonly a problem for young children after inhalation injury
- Young children have less mature renal concentrating ability
- Young children are easily fluid overloaded
- Young children are particularly susceptible to hyponatremia and cerebral edema
- Young children have higher energy needs per unit body weight
- Children tolerate long periods of inadequate nutrition poorly
- The large surface area to mass ratio makes temperature control more difficult
- Children have a thinner skin than adults
- Skin is thinner so burns are relatively deeper and donor site healing less reliable
- Children have smaller vessels than adults
- Children grow and will predictably outgrow good surgical results
- Children seem to form hypertrophic scar with greater intensity
- Pain and anxiety are more difficult to access
- School-age children have schooling needs
- Children need strong families in recovery

Children have smaller vessels than adults. Central venous and arterial lines should be of the smallest possible caliber and placed with great care. Infants and very young children have less mature renal concentrating abilities and may require more fluid per unit body weight than predicted by common formulas for successful resuscitation. However, they are very easily fluid overloaded. All administered fluids (including arterial and central venous line flushes and medication dilutents) must be considered. Young children are particularly susceptible to cerebral edema if they become hyponatremic if resuscitated with hypotonic fluids, which will cause seizures or even herniation if unaddressed. Children consume more energy per unit body weight than adults, and they are growing. They do not tolerate inadequate nutrition and should be supplemented parenterally if not tolerating enteral feedings. Their large surface area to mass ratio makes temperature control an important issue. They should be kept warm throughout hospitalization and intraoperative hypothermia must be avoided by operating room heating.

In long-term follow-up, children grow. They will outgrow your best surgical result. They therefore need ongoing contact with a multidisciplinary team to achieve optimal long-term results. Children also seem to form hypertrophic scar with greater intensity and will predictably need prolonged scar management efforts. Children have unique developmental and psychosocial needs which must be met if recovery is to be optimal. Pain and anxiety should be addressed regularly and managed in a compassionate age-appropriate fashion. Integrating recreational therapy with rehabilitation needs is tremendously effective. School-age children should have their educational needs supported and, whenever possible, should receive assistance in reintegrating with their peers in school. Children will have better outcomes if their families are supported, both during acute hospitalization and in the years that follow.

GERIATRIC CONSIDERATIONS

Older adults also bring unique physiologic issues to the burn unit (*Table 4*). Injury mechanisms frequently involve compromised mobility, dexterity, or cognition. Sometimes injuries occur during syncopal episodes that should be evaluated.

Table 4 Geriatric considerations
- Injury mechanisms more often involve compromised mobility or dexterity
- Injury mechanisms more commonly involve abuse or neglect
- Injuries may reflect an inability to safely live alone because of compromised functioning
- Injuries occur during syncopal episodes
- Resuscitation should be carefully considered if burns are very large
- Patients may have advanced directives, spouses and families, or health care proxies who should be consulted as early as possible in their care
- Older adults often do not have the physiologic reserve of the young
- Pulmonary function may be compromised by years of smoking
- Occult or overt coronary artery or peripheral vascular disease may exist
- Muscle strength, including of respiratory muscles, may be reduced
- Renal function may be compromised with greater sensitivity to nephrotoxins or hypotension
- Skin is thinner so burns are relatively deeper and donor site healing less reliable
- Older adults may live alone or have a spouse who cannot reasonably meet discharge needs
- Discharge planning may be very involved and must be started early

AUSTERE ALTERNATIVES

Burned patients the world over share the same physiology, an initial hypodynamic phase followed by a catabolic hyperdynamic phase. In the developed world, we modify this physiology through fluid resuscitation and early wound excision and closure. In the developing world, the burn disease often takes its natural course because the resources needed to intervene are simply not available. Many practitioners in the developed world infrequently see the harsh reality of overwhelming wound sepsis (7). These resource limitations mean that patients with large burns are unlikely to survive. This is a very difficult position for a practitioner to be in, making a judgment about the wisdom of expending already scarce critical care and operative resources on a patient with a large burn. However, these judgments must be made, if only by inaction. It is more difficult in patients with mid-size burns, in whom survival is possible, but septic death just as possible. Furthermore, if patients with larger burns do survive, they may accrue burn-related deformities that interfere with successful life in the harsh rural world in which they often live, without the luxury of the social supports those of us in the developed world take for granted (8).

Solutions to these dilemmas are few. I have great respect for burn care providers placed in these difficult circumstances. In some few instances, partnerships with burn programs in more developed countries may provide a partial respite from these difficult realities.

7 Wound sepsis is a common threat to life in patients managed in resource-challenged locations, where prompt wound excision is not an option.

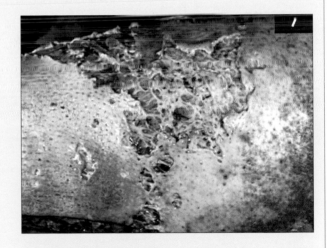

8 In austere settings, in which early excision and closure of wounds cannot be practiced, burns are often left to heal by a slow and painful process of contraction and epithelialization.

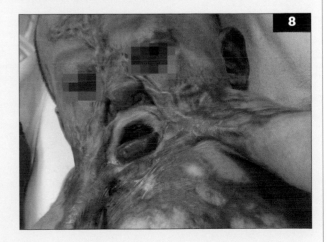

Resuscitation should be carefully considered if burns are very large, particularly in the presence of inhalation injury. Data exist suggesting that mortality is over 90% in those over 60 years of age with third-degree burns over 40% and concomitant inhalation injury. Spouses, families, and health care proxies should be consulted as early as possible in the care of such patients so that proper ethical decisions can be made. Older adults do not have the physiologic reserve of the young. Pulmonary function may be compromised by years of smoking. Occult or overt coronary artery or peripheral vascular disease may exist. Muscle strength, including that of respiratory muscles, may be reduced. Renal function may be reduced with resulting greater sensitivity to nephrotoxic drugs or hypotensive insults. The skin of the elderly person is thinner than that of the younger adult, hence full-thickness injury is more common and donor site healing is a predictable problem.

In long-term follow-up, elderly adults also have unique issues. On the positive side, hypertrophic scarring seems less intense, and the need for reconstructive surgery reduced. However, elders often live alone or have a spouse who cannot reasonably meet their discharge needs for wound care, transportation, or general support. Their children may live far away. Living alone or going back to previous living arrangements after discharge may be a poor option. Discharge planning may be very involved and must be started early.

CHAPTER 3

INITIAL CARE

'Always give a hundred percent, and you'll never have to second-guess yourself.'

Tommy John (1943– present),
26 season major-league American baseball player.

'The very first requirement in a hospital is that it should do the sick no harm.'

Florence Nightingale (1820–1910),
British nurse and humanitarian.

Triage of burn patients will vary depending on the system in which care is provided. In the developed world, where regionalization of burn care has become established, decisions must be made about who should be triaged to a burn center and who should be managed locally. The American Burn Association has developed a set of guidelines (*Table 1*) to facilitate these decisions, but in every case, clinical judgment and a knowledge of local capabilities should be paramount.

PREHOSPITAL AND INTERHOSPITAL TRANSPORT

Quality burn care begins with well-executed prehospital care and transportation. Optimally, protocols and arrangements can be set up in advance. In any case, communication between providers at the different sites facilitates smooth transportation. Transport priorities include control of the airway, secure venous access, maintenance of body temperature, fluid administration if transport time will be more than 1 hr, placement of bladder and nasogastric catheters, documentation of the events of the injury and in-transport care, and efforts to notify family members (*Table 5*). If inhalation injury is suspected, upright positioning and humidified oxygen are important initial measures.

Table 5 Acute burn transfer advice

- The airway must be adequately controlled prior to transport. Some cases may require prophylactic intubation prior to transport
- Patients with serious burns should be transported with a nasogastric tube, bladder catheter, and two well secured intravenous lines
- Fluid resuscitation should generally begin prior to transfer if transport time will exceed 1 hr
- Initial infusion for children <20 kg: D5RL at maintenance rate (approximately 4 ml/kg/hr for the first 10 kg, 2 ml/kg/hr for the next 10 kg, and 1 ml/kg/hr for weight over 20 kg) PLUS RL at 2–3 ml/kg/% burn over 1st 24 hr, 1st half in the first 8 postburn hr. Infusions should be adjusted based on urine output and vital signs
- Initial infusion for children >20 kg: RL at 2–4 ml/kg/% burn over 1st 24 hr, 1st half in the first 8 postburn hr. Infusions should be adjusted based on urine output and vital signs
- Initial infusion for adults: RL at 2–4 ml/kg/% burn over 1st 24 hr, 1st half in the first 8 postburn hr. Infusions should be adjusted based on urine output and vital signs
- Make every effort to keep patients warm during transport. Wounds should be covered with a clean, dry sheet
- Vital signs should be monitored. Pulse oximetry is ideal. Attendant skill level should be appropriate to the severity of the injury

Hypothermia is a particular threat during transport. Due to the loss of the epidermal barrier, evaporative heat loss can be extreme. Hypothermia is easier prevented than treated, particularly in small children (**9**). Transporting vehicles and emergency department receiving areas should be warmed prior to patient arrival. Initial dressing should be dry clean sheets rather than wet. Immediate cooling of a wound involving less than 15% of the body surface may help limit burn depth, but by the time emergency response personnel have arrived, this brief window of opportunity is usually gone.

PRIMARY SURVEY

Although many patients are quite hemodynamically stable for the first 1–2 hr, the first encounter with a patient who has suffered serious burn can be disturbing enough to interfere with organized thinking. To facilitate proper performance in such circumstances, an organized approach has been developed by the American Burn Association through its Advanced Burn Life Support Course, available in both a classroom and online format (www.ameriburn.org). The evaluation should begin with a primary survey. The primary survey, taught as part of the Advanced Trauma Life Support Course of the American College of Surgeons' Committee on Trauma (see Textbox: The ATLS concept), involves a rapid assessment of the airway, breathing, circulatory state, neurologic status, and external appearace of the patient. During the primary survey, any immediately

life-threatening problems are identified and addressed. In burn patients, these generally include an unstable airway and the absence of vascular access. Burn patients tend to be reasonably stable for the first 1–2 hr after injury, allowing a more studied approach to these priorities in many situations.

Ensuring a stable controlled airway is the highest priority part of the primary survey. The airways of burn patients, particularly young patients, can be among the most challenging of airways to manage. If patients display signs of impending airway obstruction from edema, they should be intubated. If they are at risk for airway obstruction, demonstrating stridor or retractions, particularly if a long transport is imminent, they should be intubated. If the airway is likely to be safe, the risks of intubation are not justified. This difficult clinical decision can be made in consultation with the receiving facility. Given the challenging nature of airway control in this setting, it is optimal if the most experienced people available are called upon to participate in initial efforts to secure these airways. Further, it is absolutely essential that the endotrachael tube be properly secured to prevent the potential catastrophe of accidental extubation. Security and position of the tube should be monitored as the most important vital sign (**10**). On occasion, young children may aspirate hot liquids and develop life-threatening upper airway edema requiring intubation. A history of coughing and gagging along with perioral burns suggests the diagnosis (**11**).

Reliable vascular access is an essential component of early management of patients with serious burns. Peripheral access is often difficult in cold, hypovolemic

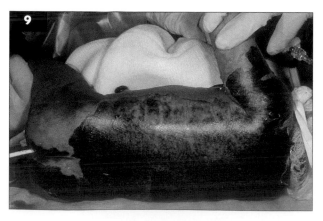

9 Virtually all patients with extensive loss of the epidermal barrier will become hypothermic during transport if this is not anticipated.

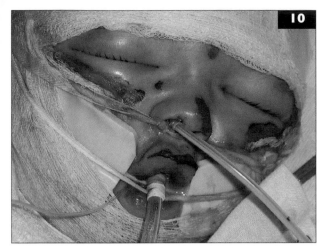

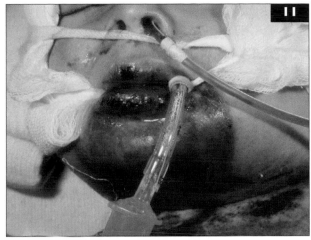

10 A tie-harness works well to secure the endotracheal tube. Tube security should be frequently reassessed to minimize the chance of catastrophic unplanned extubation.

11 Hot liquids are occasionally aspirated by young children and can cause severe swelling of the upper airway. This child demonstrates a typical pattern, with perioral burning.

THE ATLS CONCEPT

The Advanced Trauma Life Support (ATLS) paradigm was initially conceived by an American orthopedic surgeon and pilot, James Styner, after he survived a horrific plane crash in 1976 in which his wife was killed and three children seriously injured. He felt the care his family received at the nearby rural Nebraska hospital was chaotic and ineffective and he decided to do something about it. With a group of Nebraska surgeons and educators, assisted by the state university, a set of materials to teach organized initial trauma care was developed and taught the following year. These courses became the scaffold leading to the ATLS course promulgated by the American College of Surgeons' Committee on Trauma, beginning in the early 1980s. The training program has been adopted in over 40 countries, and is generally known in Europe and is mandatory for trauma staff in the UK*. Initial care of seriously injured patients is difficult. Providers can be overwhelmed by numerous immediate priorities that conflict with one another. Clear thinking is difficult. The goal of the ATLS program is to teach providers an organized approach to a chaotic problem. The course has been exceptionally successful, and tens of thousands of providers now use its approach. Multiple studies have documented its efficacy. Organized thinking works. Thousands of lives have been saved. This scaffold was then used to develop the Advanced Burn Life Support Course, which is available as a classroom or on-line experience through the American Burn Association.

*Many countries, including the UK, The Netherlands, South Africa, and Malaysia, also run the Emergency Management of Severe Burns (EMSB) course. This course is similar to, and can be taught in conjuction with, the ATLS program. The course was originally developed by the Australian and New Zealand Burn Association.

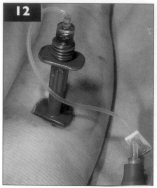

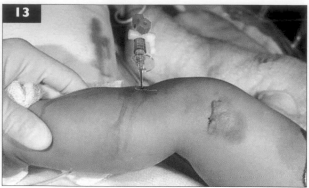

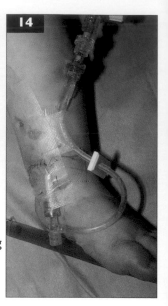

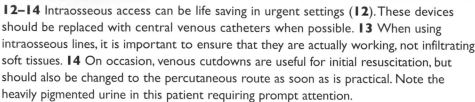

12–14 Intraosseous access can be life saving in urgent settings (**12**). These devices should be replaced with central venous catheters when possible. **13** When using intraosseous lines, it is important to ensure that they are actually working, not infiltrating soft tissues. **14** On occasion, venous cutdowns are useful for initial resuscitation, but should also be changed to the percutaneous route as soon as is practical. Note the heavily pigmented urine in this patient requiring prompt attention.

patients, especially small children. In this setting, intraosseous access may be useful (**12**). Dedicated intraosseous catheters are optimal, but heavy spinal needles may also be placed. When using intraosseous access, it is important to ensure that they are actually working, not infiltrating soft tissues (**13**). Venous cutdowns can be useful when other methods are not available (**14**). Ideally, central venous access is secured early during care of most patients with serious burns.

BURN-SPECIFIC SECONDARY SURVEY

Initial evaluation of the wound is described in Chapter 5. Burn patients are prone to a number of characteristic problems and complications in the early hours and days after injury (*Table 6*). Knowledge of these common traps facilitates anticipation and prompt management, minimizing their associated morbidity. A burn-specific secondary survery, analogous to the trauma secondary survey of the Advanced Trauma Life Support Course is a useful tool in this regard, and should be applied to all patients with serious burns.

An accurate understanding of the mechanism of injury is important, but surprisingly difficult to come by when patients are transferred over a substantial distance. A directed effort, often through phone calls to referring emergency departments or family members, will provide valuable information when making decisions about additional imaging for trauma or special monitoring and management

considerations for comorbid conditions.

A good ocular exam is an important part of the secondary survey, and becomes more difficult as facial edema worsens. In patients with deep facial burns and large overall surface burns, retrobulbar edema may result in vision-threatening intraocular hypertension. In patients at risk, intraocular pressure should be measured. If elevated, lateral canthotomy can be done at the bedside to decompress the orbit (**15**). Other ocular injuries should be noted, including corneal

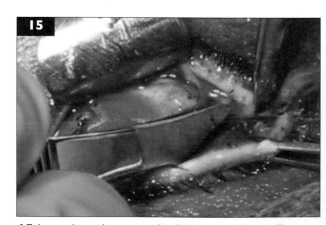

15 Lateral canthotomy, a bedside procedure, will effectively decompress the orbit in the setting of critically elevated intraocular pressure due to retrobulbar edema.

Table 6 Burn-specific secondary survey highlights

History

- Document mechanism of injury, closed space exposure, extrication time, delay in seeking attention, fluid given during transport, and prior illnesses and injuries

HEENT

- The globes should be examined and corneal epithelium stained with fluorescein before adnexal swelling makes examination difficult. Adnexal swelling provides excellent coverage and protection of the globe during the first days after injury, so tarsorrhaphy is virtually never indicated acutely
- Corneal epithelial loss can be overt, giving a clouded appearance to the cornea, but is more often subtle, requiring fluorescein staining for documentation. Topical ophthalmic antibiotics constitute optimal initial treatment
- Intraocular hypertension should be excluded in patients with large burns including the face
- Signs of airway involvement include perioral and intraoral burns or carbonaceous material and progressive hoarseness
- Hot liquid can be aspirated in conjunction with a facial scald injury and result in acute airway compromise requiring urgent intubation
- Endotracheal tube security is crucial and is best maintained with an umbilical tape harness, rather than adhesive tape, on the burned face

Neck

- Radiographic evaluation is driven by the mechanism of injury
- Rarely, in patients with very deep burns, neck escharotomies are needed to facilitate venous drainage of the head

Cardiac

- The cardiac rhythm should be monitored for 24–72 hr in those with high-voltage electrical injury
- If intravascular volume and oxygenation are adequately supported, significant arrhythmias are unusual in otherwise healthy patients

Pulmonary

- Optimize chest wall compliance by performing liberal chest escharotomies when needed
- Severe inhalation injury may lead to slough of endobronchial mucosa and thick endobronchial secretions that can occlude the endotracheal tube, so one should be prepared for sudden endotracheal tube occlusions

Vascular

- The perfusion of burned extremities should be vigilantly monitored by serial examinations. Indications for escharotomy include decreasing temperature, increasing consistency, slowed capillary refill and diminished Doppler flow in the digital vessels. One should not wait until flow in named vessels is compromised to decompress the extremity
- Fasciotomy is indicated after electrical or deep thermal injury when distal flow is compromised on clinical examination. Compartment pressures can be helpful, but clinically worrisome extremities should be decompressed regardless of compartment pressure readings

Abdomen

- Nasogastric tubes should be in place and their function verified, especially before air transport in unpressurized helicopters
- An inappropriate resuscitative volume requirement may be a sign of an occult intra-abdominal injury
- Torso escharotomies may be required to facilitate ventilation in the presence of deep circumferential abdominal wall burns
- Immediate ulcer prophylaxis with histamine receptor blockers and antacids is indicated in all patients with serious burns

Genitourinary

- Bladder catheterization facilitates using urinary output as a resuscitation endpoint and is appropriate in all patients who require a fluid resuscitation
- It is important to ensure that the foreskin is reduced over the bladder catheter after insertion, as progressive swelling may otherwise result in paraphimosis

Neurologic

- An early neurologic evaluation is important, as the patient's sensorium is often progressively compromised by medication or hemodynamic instability during the hours after injury. This may require CT scanning in those with a mechanism of injury consistent with head trauma
- Pain and anxiety medication should be administered within the bounds of safety
- Patients who require neuromuscular blockade for transport should also receive adequate sedation and analgesia

Extremities

- Extremities that are at risk for ischemia, particularly those with circumferential thermal burns or those with electrical injury, should be dressed so they can be frequently examined
- Tense extremities should be decompressed promptly by escharotomy and/or fasciotomy when clinical examination reveals increasing consistency, decreasing temperature, and diminished Doppler flow in digital vessels

Continued overleaf

Table 6 Burn-specific secondary survey highlights (*continued*)

- The need for escharotomy usually becomes evident during the early hours of resuscitation. Therefore, most escharotomies can be delayed until transport has been effected if transport times will not extend beyond 6 hr after injury
- Burned extremities should be elevated and splinted in a position of function

Wound

- Wounds, although often underestimated in depth and overestimated in size on initial examination, should be evaluated for size, depth, and the presence of circumferential components
- Burn wounds are potentially tetanus prone, and tetanus immune status should be determined and appropriately supplemented

Laboratory

- Arterial blood gas analysis is important when airway compromise or inhalation injury is present
- A normal admission carboxyhemoglobin concentration does not eliminate the possibility of a significant exposure as the half-life of carboxyhemoblobin is 30–40 min in those effectively ventilated with 100% oxygen
- Baseline hemoglobin and electrolytes can be helpful later during resuscitation

Radiography

- The radiographic evaluation is driven by the mechanism of injury and the need to document placement of lines and tubes

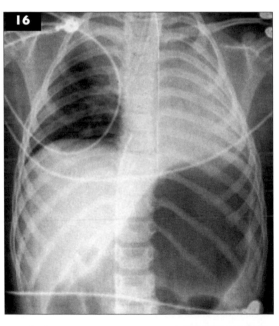

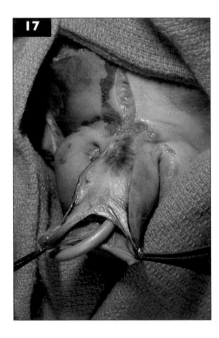

16 Acute gastric dilatation can compromise ventilation and increase the risk of aspiration. Note the simultaneous presence of a right mainstem intubation with collapse of the left lung.

17 Deeply burned male genitalia may make it difficult to cannulate the bladder, which can be facilitated by dorsal slit of a deeply burned foreskin.

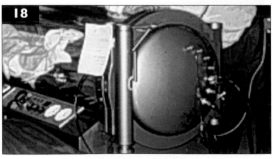

18 Hyperbaric oxygen therapy can be administered to patients requiring mechanical ventilation. Wheezing, air-trapping, mucous plugging, and hemodynamic lability are relative contraindictations.

burns (most common) and hyphema.

Inhalation injury is a diagnosis best made by history and physical exam, supplemented with bronchoscopy in occasional cases. Most patients with inhalation injury have a normal chest X-ray and pulmonary function initially, except for the common occurrence of bronchospasm, which is usually well-managed with nebulized beta-agonists. Typically, 3–7 days later, as they slough damaged endo-bronchial epithelium, respiratory compromise develops. It is wise to take advantage of this common early window of good pulmonary function to perform large initial excisions or to effect transport to a site of definitive care, as both are more risky during acute pulmonary deterioration.

Acute gastric dilatation can compromise ventilation and increase the risk of aspiration (16). It is effectively managed with nasogastric decompression. Deeply burned male genitalia may make it difficult to cannulate the bladder, which can be facilitated by dorsal slit of a deeply burned foreskin (17). Some patients with inhalation injury will suffer concomitant carbon monoxide intoxication. Current literature is divided on the efficacy of hyperbaric oxygen treatment. The standard of care for significant carbon monoxide exposure is 6 hr of 100% normobaric oxygen. Hyperbaric oxygen treatments are reasonable in stable patients if locally available (18). Wheezing, air-trapping, mucous plugging, and hemodynamic lability are relative contraindictations.

INITIAL WOUND CARE

Burn wounds are very clean initially, essentially sterilized by the injury. It is only in the hours and days following injury that bacteria proliferate in the avascular eschar. During transport and initial evaluation, wounds are best kept dry and covered with a sterile sheet. Later, topical agents, or occasionally temporary membranes, are applied to decrease vapor loss, prevent desiccation, and slow bacterial growth. There are an increasing number of substances available (*Table 7,* overleaf). Various preparations of silver sulfadiazine, an opaque white cream, are painless on application, have fair to poor eschar penetration, have no metabolic side-effects, and have a broad antibacterial spectrum. Mafenide acetate, as an 11% cream or 5% solution, can be uncomfortable on application, is a carbonic anhydrase inhibitor, has excellent eschar penetration, and a broad antibacterial spectrum (although it does not

cover fungi). Silver is an extremely effective topical agent and is generally applied as aqueous 0.5% silver nitrate, which is painless on application, has poor eschar penetration, leaches electrolytes, but has a broad spectrum of activity (including fungi), and can be used on adjacent wounds, grafts, and donor sites. Silver impregnated membranes, such as Acticoat® (Smith & Nephew, Hull, UK) and Aquacel-Ag® (Convatec, Princeton, NJ) are also useful in selected wounds (see *Table 12,* page 43).

Burns are tetanus prone wounds. Tetanus status should be documented and supplemented if indicated. If in doubt, active immunization should be administered. In those who are not immunized or who have incomplete or questionable tetanus immune status, passive immunization is advisable. This is particularly true if burns are extensive, deep, chronic, or contaminated.

ESCHAROTOMIES AND FASCIOTOMIES

Extremity perfusion and torso compliance can be compromised quite severely by progressive soft tissue edema during burn resuscitation. Limb salvage, ventilation, and renal perfusion may depend upon timely escharotomy and/or fasciotomy. Extremities at risk for ischemia from subeschar edema should be carefully monitored for perfusion. Perfusion pressures at the soft tissue level are less than one-third of those in named vessels. Endpoints for perfusion should not be palpable pulses. Rather, tissue turgor, temperature, Doppler flow in digital pulp, capillary refill, and transmission oximetry should be monitored in extremities at risk.

In most patients, escharotomies can be performed at the bedside using coagulating electrocautery to minimize blood loss. On the extremities, axially oriented medial and lateral incisions can be made to section the deep eschar while avoiding exposure or injury to underlying superficial structures. Superficial structures most at risk during extremity escharotomy are the trachea, brachial artery in the upper arm, ulnar nerve at the elbow, superficial peroneal nerve at the knee, and the neurovascular bundles and extensors of the digits.

When contemplating escharotomies of the hands and digits, the arm and forearm should first be decompressed. Often this will result in adequate flow to the digits (which can be detected with a Doppler probe on the digital pulp). If proximal decom-

Table 7 Common topical wound medications and membranes in out-patient use

Silver sulfadiazene:
- Broad antibacterial spectrum
- Painless on application
- Moderately expensive

Mafenide acetate (11% cream or 5% solution):
- Broad antibacterial spectrum
- Penetrates eschar including cartilage
- Carbonic anhydrase inhibitor
- Cream uncomfortable on application

(Not generally available in the UK)

Petrolatum (paraffin gauze, Tulle gause):
- Bland and nontoxic
- Occlusive ointment
- Improves pain control
- No antibacterial activity
- Inexpensive

Various debriding enzymes:
- Variable use for deep dermal wounds
- May increase rate of spontaneous slough and re-epithelialization
- Use is highly program-dependent

(Not commonly used for outpatients)

Various antibiotic ointments:
- Viscous nonstaining carrier
- Little penetration
- Selected spectrum
- Occlusive ointment
- Improves pain control
- Inexpensive

(In the UK, not often used in outpatients)

Porcine xenograft (Brennen Medical Inc., St. Paul, MN):
- Biologic membrane that adheres to coagulum
- Excellent pain control
- Small risk of submembrane fluid collections
- Must be followed for submembrane infection
- Moderately expensive

(In the UK, not often used in outpatients)

Biobrane (Dow–Hickham, Sugarland, TX):
- Bilaminate synthetic membrane
- Fibrovascular ingrowth into inner layer
- Good pain control
- Risk of submembrane fluid collections
- Should be followed for submembrane infection

(In the UK, not often used in outpatients)

Aquacel-Ag (Convatec, Princeton, NJ):
- Absorptive hydrofiber
- Delivers low concentrations of silver
- Should be followed for submembrane infection

Acticoat (Smith & Nephew, Hull, UK):
- Nonadherent occlusive membrane
- Delivers low concentrations of silver to the wound
- Should be followed for submembrane infection

Various semipermeable membranes:
- Provide vapor and bacterial barrier
- Facilitate pain control
- Risk of submembrane fluid collections
- Should be followed for submembrane infection

Various hydrocolloid dressings:
- Provide vapor and bacterial barrier
- Facilitate pain control
- Absorb exudate

Various impregnated gauzes:
- Provide partial vapor barrier
- Facilitate pain control
- Inexpensive
- Allow drainage

Note: in the UK, glycerol-preserved allografts (Euro Skin Bank, NL) are preferred for a biological dressing

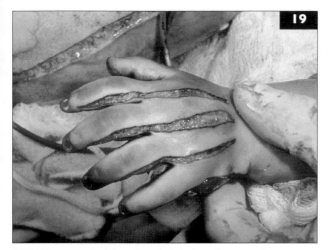

19 When needed, hand and digital escharotomies can be safely performed with a single axial incision on the ulnar aspect of the digits and the radial aspect of the thumb, protecting the more important innervation of the opposing surfaces of the digits. The incisions on the ulnar aspect of the central three digits can be extended onto the dorsum of the hand, between the extensors, to facilitate complete decompression of the hand.

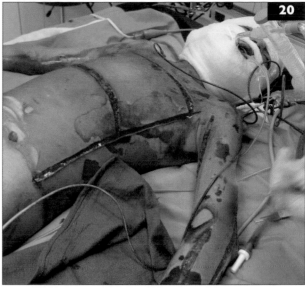

20 Difficulty with ventilation, increasing inflating pressures, and a falling urine output may respond to decompression of the torso. Incisions can be made along the mid-axillary lines and connected across the mid-line.

pression does not adequately improve digital flow, a single axial incision can be made on the ulnar aspect of the digits and the radial aspect of the thumb, protecting the more important innervation of the opposing surfaces of the digits. The incisions on the ulnar aspect of the central three digits can be extended onto the dorsum of the hand, between the extensors, to facilitate complete decompression of the hand (**19**).

Extremity fasciotomies, usually the forearm and/or leg, are sometimes required in the setting of high-voltage injury or very deep thermal burn (see **4, 5**). Complete upper extremity fasciotomy often requires both volar and dorsal forearm incisions, widely opening fascia encompassing individual muscle bundles, opening the carpal tunnel, and dorsal hand fasciotomy. Several incisions are recommended. The curvilinear incision illustrated in **4, 5** allows access to individual muscle bundles in the volar forearm, to decompress the carpal tunnel through a contiguous incision, and creates a vascularized flap of skin to maintain coverage over the median nerve at the wrist. However, separate, simple longitudinal incisions also suffice. On the

dorsal aspect of the arm, straight linear incisions are adequate. Intermetacarpal incisions on the hand allow decompression of the intrinsic muscles of the hand. The four compartments of the leg are ideally decompressed using medial and lateral incisions which can be done through well-designed escharotomy incisions. If extremity decompression is not performed when needed, late functional deficits will result. On occasion, late sepsis may develop in necrotic compartments.

Decompression of the torso may be needed in the setting of deep circumferential, or near circumferential, torso burns. Symptoms include progressive difficulty with ventilation, increasing inflating pressures, and a falling urine output if renal blood flow is compromised. Intraabdominal pressures can be followed by transducing bladder pressure, with unacceptable increases defined as between 25 and 30 mmHg. Escharotomy incisions can be made along the mid-axillary lines and connected across the mid-line (**20**). In some infrequent cases, usually in the setting of delayed resuscitation of a very large burn, visceral edema occurs to the degree that abdominal compartment syndrome results. In this situation, escharotomy does not relieve intra-abdominal hypertension and laparotomy with creation of a temporary loose closure is required (**21**). Ideally, the

abdomen is closed within 5 days, often facilitated by component release of the abdominal fascia. If torso decompression is not performed when needed, renal failure, bowel necrosis, and respiratory failure can result.

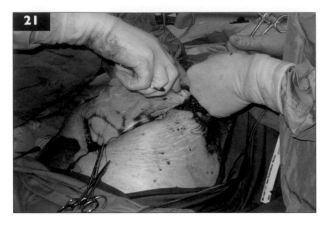

21 Infrequently, visceral edema occurs to the degree that abdominal compartment syndrome results, and escharotomy does not relieve intra-abdominal hypertension. Laparotomy with creation of a temporary loose closure is required. This can be done in the ICU.

AUSTERE ALTERNATIVES: INITIAL CARE

In the austere environment, an initial decision must be made regarding the wisdom of an attempt at resuscitation (**22**). Ideally, these decisions are made as a group, thoughtfully, and well in advance of specific incidents. Critical components of the decision are available resources both for acute care and for later reconstruction. These decisions will differ when large numbers of patients are received in disaster scenarios. When attempting resuscitation in an austere environment or in the midst of a disaster involving large numbers of patients, details of initial evaluation and fluid resuscitation are modified based on resource availability. For example, if there is no colloid available for infusion, then none can be administered, and a pure crystalloid resuscitation is required. If central venous lines are impractical, peripheral lines or cut-downs may be required. If mechanical ventilation is not practical, those requiring intubation may not be intubated, unless interunit relationships exist that would allow such patients to be transported to a higher level of care. In some settings, care of patients with very large burns is impractical and burn sizes at which resuscitation is not done should be agreed upon. These decisions can never be easy, but it is optimal if these scenarios are discussed before individual incidents occur, to allow for proper planning and to take the decision-making load off involved individual providers.

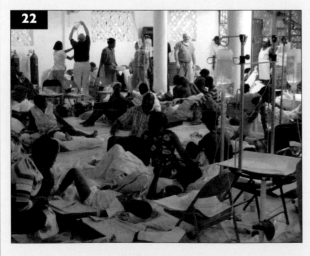

22 In most parts of the world, resource constraints impact on care decisions on a daily basis. These allocatioin issues are magnified during disasters, such as during the 2010 Haiti earthquake.

CHAPTER 4

FLUID RESUSCITATION

'Success in any endeavor requires single-minded attention to detail.'
Willie Sutton (1901–1980), bank robber.

'Simplicity is the ultimate sophistication.'
Leonardo da Vinci (1452–1519),
Italian Renaissance man.

Before effective burn resuscitation formulas were developed, it was rare for patients with burns in excess of 40% of the body surface to survive long enough to die of wound sepsis. However, successful burn resuscitation can only be loosely guided by formulas. The varying recommendations of existing burn resuscitation formulas highlight the critical importance of regular assessment of age-specific endpoints during resuscitation. There is no formula that will accurately predict the volume requirements of an individual patient. Therefore, it is essential to have an interested presence by the bedside throughout these often inconvenient hours, adjusting volume infusions frequently, if one is to achieve reliably optimal outcomes.

RESUSCITATION PHYSIOLOGY

The knowledge that burn patients required additional fluid was only grasped in the 1930s and 1940s after physicians were faced with large numbers of burn casualties in civilian disasters such as the Rialto Concert Hall and Cocoanut Grove fires, and during the war years (see Textbox: Clifford Johnson's resuscitation). In the following decades, numerous burn resuscitation formulas based on burn and body size were developed, although none was always

---

CLIFFORD JOHNSON'S RESUSCITATION

Perhaps the most acclaimed patient from the November 1942 Cocoanut Grove fire was a young Coast Guard sailor, Clifford Johnson (**23**), who was on a blind date to the Cocoanut Grove nightclub on the night of the disaster. He initially escaped the burning building, but went back inside to find his date (who had already escaped). He suffered a 40% flame burn and was taken to Boston City Hospital, along with hundreds of other casualties. By the standards of that time, his injury was not survivable. Given the hopelessness of his case, he was initially placed under the care of a young medical student, Phillip Butler. Based on his clinical impressions, Mr. Butler (who later became an internist)

Continued overleaf

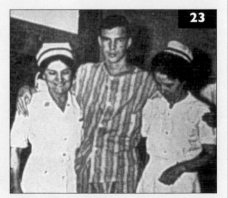

23 Clifford Johnson, celebrated survivor of the Cocoanut Grove Fire, towards the end of his hospitalization.

administered amounts of fluid far in excess of the then-current standard of care (but close to what would later be recommended by the Parkland Formula decades later).

Surprisingly to all, Mr. Johnson survived burn shock under Mr. Butler's care. Then ensued a nightmarish experience of recurrent shock, florid wound sepsis, poorly controlled pain, ineffective topical wound therapy, early use of intravenous albumin, primitive surgical techniques, graft failure, narcotic addiction, grinding hard work and compassion of providers, and ultimate survival, all wrenchingly described by Paul Benzaquin in his classic book on the Cocoanut Grove Fire. The clinical course of Clifford Johnson is one of the few detailed lay descriptions of the natural history of a large burn, and illustrates how far we have come in only a few decades. Unfortunately, similar stories still occur today in less developed parts of the world, usually with fatal outcomes.

accurate. A universally accurate burn resuscitation formula is inherently impossible, as in addition to burn and body size, resuscitation needs vary with burn depth, wound vapor transmission characteristics, resuscitation timing, burn mechanism, inhalation injury, and other individual variables. This emphasizes the importance of ongoing monitoring and frequent infusion titration during resuscitation.

Although the fundamental biology of burn shock remains poorly understood, the clinical consequences are very well described. The first 12–36 hours are characterized by a hypodynamic state, with reduced cardiac output and temperature. Reduced circulating volume is a result of transeschar fluid loss and a cryptic, but clinically dramatic, diffuse loss of capillary integrity resulting in impressive diffuse soft tissue edema (**24**). In patients with larger burns, this 'ebb phase' must be supported with intravascular volume, or death will result. Subsequently, a hyperdynamic state, with increased cardiac output and muscle catabolism develops. In patients with larger burns, this 'flow phase' must be supported with nutrition and wound closure, or death will eventually result. Exactly how burn shock during the ebb phase should be addressed remains controversial. The ideal fluid resuscitation formula has yet to be developed. The wild variation in the specific recommendations of formulas in common use highlights the importance of frequent bedside assessment of age-specific endpoints throughout the resuscitation period, with frequent adjustment of infusion rates to balance individual changes in physiology (*Table 8*). There is no formula that will predict the needs of an individual patient.

RESUSCITATION PRACTICE

Common resuscitation formulas differ in their recommendations on the amount of isotonic crystalloid, free water, and colloid administration. Most formulas recommend that all crystalloid be isotonic during the first 24 hr, generally Ringer's

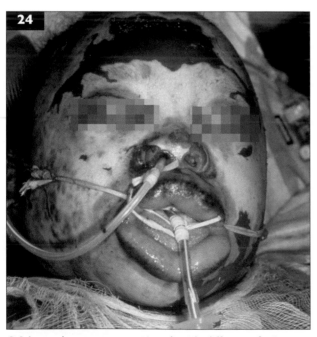

24 Large burns are associated with diffuse soft tissue edema. Edema involving the face and pharynx can threaten the airway. Careful attention to endotrachael tube security is important in this setting.

lactate (RL) solution, as this avoids the hyper-chloremic acidosis that can be seen with large saline infusions. A commonly advocated consensus formula is presented in *Table 9*. A 3% hypertonic saline resuscitation was advocated by some authors in the 1980s, as it was associated with reduced soft tissue edema. This practice has generally been abandoned because hypertonic resuscitation is technically challenging and has been shown to increase mortality in at least one study. A slightly hypertonic solution made by adding sodium bicarbonate to RL solution is felt to be useful by some practitioners, particularly in pediatric resuscitation.

The gluconeogenetic capacity of older children and adolescents is such that no glucose containing solutions are required during resuscitation. In infants and younger children hypoglycemia is a threat, and RL with 5% dextrose (D5RL) should be administered at a maintenance rate of approximately 4 ml/kg/hr for the first 10 kg of body weight,

---

Table 8 Typical resuscitation targets
- **Sensorium:** arouseable and comfortable
- **Temperature:** warm centrally and peripherally
- **Systolic blood pressure:** for infants, 60 mmHg systolic; for older children, 70–90 + 2× age in years mmHg; for adults, mean arterial pressure >60 mmHg
- **Pulse:** 80–180/min (age dependent), easily palpable peripherally
- **Urine output:** 0.5–1 ml/kg/hr (glucose negative)
- **Base deficit:** <2

Table 9 A consensus resuscitation formula
FIRST 24 HR
Adults and children >20kg:
> **Ringer's lactate:** 2–4 ml/kg/% burn/24 hr (first half in first 8 hr)
> **Colloid*:** none, but many practitioners would advise 5% albumin at 1× maintenance rate if burn is >40% TBSA

Children <20kg:
> **Ringer's lactate:** 2–3 ml/kg/% burn/24 hr (first half in first 8 hr)
> **Ringer's lactate with 5% dextrose:** maintenance rate (approximately 4 ml/kg/hr for the first 10 kg, 2 ml/kg/hr for the next 10 kg, and 1 ml/kg/hr for weight >20 kg)
> **Colloid*:** none, but many practitioners would advise 5% albumin at 1× maintenance rate if burn is >40% TBSA

SECOND 24 HR
All patients:
> **Crystalloid:** To maintain urine output, commonly requiring approximately 1.5× maintenance rate. If silver nitrate is used, sodium leaching will mandate continued isotonic crystalloid. If another topical agent is used, free water requirement is significant. Serum sodium should be monitored closely. Nutritional support should begin, ideally by the enteral route.
> **Colloid*: (5% albumin in Ringer's lactate to maintain serum albumin at or above 2.0 g/dl [20 g/l]):**
> 0–30% burn: none   50–70% burn: 0.4 ml/kg/% burn/24 hr
> 30–50% burn: 0.3 ml/kg/% burn/24 hr   70–100% burn: 0.5 ml/kg/% burn/24 hr

* The role of colloid in burn resuscitation is an area of controversy. Check with the program to which the patient will be referred for their recommendations. This author routinely administers 5% albumin at a maintenance rate to patients with burns >40% of the TBSA, beginning immediately.

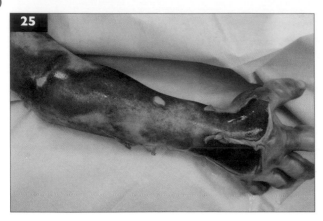

25 Extremities at risk for ischemia from subeschar edema should be carefully monitored for perfusion. Perfusion pressures at the soft tissue level are less than one-third of mean blood pressure in bigger named vessels. Endpoints for perfusion should not be palpable pulses. Rather, tissue turgor, temperature, Doppler flow in digital pulp, capillary refill, and transmission oximetry should be monitored in extremities at risk. Ischemia will generally not present until well into resuscitation.

2 ml/kg/hr for the next 10 kg, and 1 ml/kg/hr for weight over 20 kg.

Burns less than 15% of the body surface generally are not associated with the extensive diffuse capillary leak that larger burns are. Patients with burns in this size range can be managed with fluid administered at 150% of a calculated maintenance rate, and close observation of the status of their hydration, weighing the diapers of younger children. Those who are able and willing to take fluid by mouth may be given fluid by mouth with additional fluid given by IV at a maintenance rate.

Even in well-controlled resuscitations, total extravascular water will increase. The clinical consequences include limb threatening ischemia in areas of circumferential eschar, reduced ventilation if there is circumferential torso eschar, and worsening of intracompartmental edema in those with high-voltage injuries or very deep thermal extremity burns. These areas need to be closely watched during resuscitation so that appropriate and timely decompression procedures can be performed (**25**).

Pigmented urine is commonly seen in patients with high-voltage electrical or very deep thermal injury (**26**). To avoid renal tubular injury, pigment should be recognized and cleared promptly. This can generally be accomplished by infusion of additional crystalloid to the endpoint of a urine output of 2 ml/kg/hr. The administration of bicarbonate may hinder pigment entry into the tubular cells. In rare circumstances, mannitol is a reasonable adjunct, but its use obscures urine output as an important

resuscitation endpoint. It is always important to ensure that bladder catheters are not obstructed in patients with worrisome low urine outputs (**27**).

The timing, amount, and type of colloid administration for optimal burn resuscitation remain controversial. Most formulas developed in the 1960s–1990s recommended little or no colloid in the first 24 hr. However, in more recent decades, many practitioners (including this author) have noted a clinically important reduction in volume requirements in patients with large burns when colloid is administered early. Over-resuscitation seems more common with pure crystalloid resuscitations, and carries significant potential morbidity (**28, 29**). This author routinely administers 5% albumin at a maintenance rate during the first 24 hr of resuscitation in patients with greater than 40% TBSA burns, beginning from the time of injury, and continuing for 24–48 hours. Serum albumin levels are monitored with the goal of maintaining them at or above 2.0 g/dl (20 g/l), to support colloid oncotic pressure; 5% albumin is heat-treated and carries very little risk. This seems to result in less soft tissue edema and pulmonary dysfunction. However, it is important to emphasize that there is currently no uniformly accepted practice in this area.

After 18–24 hr, capillary integrity generally returns to normal in well-resuscitated patients. Fluid requirements decrease and fluid administration should be reduced. This can be done in a timely and effective way if resuscitation endpoints have been frequently monitored. In most patients, even those

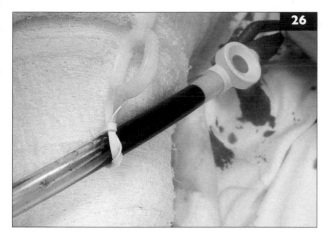

26 Pigmented urine is commonly seen with very deep thermal burns or high-voltage injuries. It should be cleared promptly.

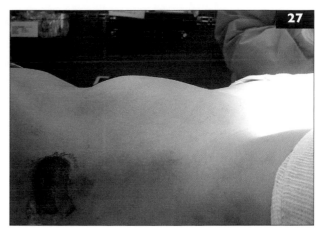

27 Unrecognized obstruction of the bladder catheter can lead to over-administration of fluid. In this patient, massive bladder distention, seen in the lateral view, is a result of unrecognized bladder catheter obstruction.

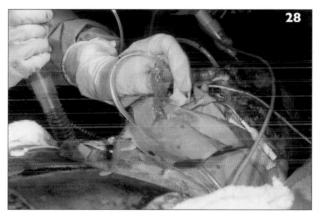

28 Over-resuscitation has led to pulmonary edema, with 'pink froth' being suctioned from the endotrachael tube.

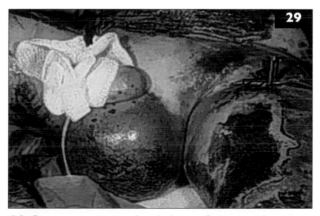

29 Over-resuscitation has led to soft tissue edema, which increases the likelihood of compartment syndromes.

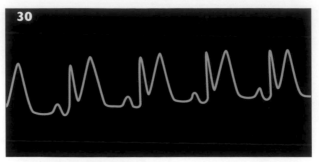

30 Over-administration of potassium, in an effort to correct hypokalemia, can lead to dangerous cardiac arrhythmias. These are often preceded by large peaked T-waves in the ECG, as demonstrated by this patient. The problem was picked up and corrected before asystole occurred.

with large burns, total fluid infusions of about 150% of maintenance suffice after 24 hr.

As fluid infusions are reduced, the wound has an increasing influence on the electrolyte picture. Wounds treated with nonaqueous topical agents generate a free water requirement, as evaporative transeschar water loss can be substantial enough to cause hypernatremia. Wounds treated with aqueous topical agents may be associated with electrolyte leaching and secondary hyponatremia. Extreme hypernatremia can be associated with intracranial bleeding. Extreme hyponatremia can cause cerebral edema and seizures. Rapid correction of hyponatremia may cause central pontine demyelinating lesions. Significant hypokalemia and hypophospha-

temia are common during the first days following resuscitation. While these should be monitored and supplemented, it is important not to overcorrect; overcorrection of hypokalemia is particularly dangerous, as it can lead to dangerous cardiac arrhythmias (**30**), including asystole. It is important to anticipate and ameliorate electrolyte shifts to minimize extreme variations in their concentrations.

While compensating for the loss of capillary integrity associated with a large burn, current resuscitation practices do not modify this physiology. There continues to be substantial research in the area, particularly with antioxidants, such as vitamin C. However, current data are insufficient to recommend this practice as a standard.

AUSTERE ALTERNATIVES: FLUID RESUSCITATION

In austere settings, intravenous resuscitation may require placement of peripheral lines or cutdowns, if central venous access is not practical. For small and mid-size burns, enteral resuscitation with electrolyte-containing solutions, such as WHO's oral rehydration solution, is an important alternative. Fluid choice is often limited, and colloid infrequently available. Monitoring of resuscitation must be by clinical exam, looking at urine output, extremity perfusion, and temperature. Advanced hemodynamic monitoring devices are usually not an option.

CHAPTER 5

WOUND EXCISION AND CLOSURE

'I dressed him. God healed him ('Je le pansai. Dieu le guérit').'

> Ambroise Paré (1517–1590), French pioneering battlefield surgeon, surgical innovator and scholar, Great Official Royal Surgeon for French Kings Henry II, Francis II, Charles IX, and Henry III.

'The best surgeon, like the best general, is he who makes the fewest mistakes.'

> Sir Astley Paston Cooper (1768–1841), British surgeon.

Clifford Johnson's story reminds us that the natural history of large burns is florid wound sepsis, multiple organ failure, and death in those that survive burn shock. Early identification, excision, and closure of full-thickness wounds changes this natural history in a profound way. Although sepsis and other complications remain common, survival and outcomes are clearly improved when the physiologic burden of necrotic tissue is promptly addressed. Wound sepsis and systemic inflammation are minimized, and hospital stays are truncated. Treatment is less agonizing, for both patients and providers. In the early years of acute burn excisional surgery (1970s and 1980s), the operations were associated with massive blood loss and extreme physiologic stress. The operations tended to be more ablative than today. Numerous techniques now exist to ameliorate these negatives. When properly performed, acute burn operations are very well tolerated, even by critically ill patients.

EVALUATION OF THE WOUND

Decisions regarding out-patient care, hospitalization, transfer, operative timing, and operation planning

depend on wound evaluation. The wound should be examined for size, depth, and circumferential components (*Table 10*).

Table 10 Initial wound evaluation: size, depth, circumferential components

Burn wound size

Lund–Browder chart: An age-specific chart that accounts for the changing body proportions with age. This is the preferred method of determining burn extent

Rule-of-Nines: A rough estimate that assumes adult body proportions. The head and neck are roughly 9%, the anterior and posterior chest are 9% each, the anterior and posterior abdomen (including buttocks) are 9% each, each upper extremity is 9%, each thigh is 9%, each leg and foot is 9%, and the remaining 1% represents the genitals

Palmar surface of the hand: The palmar surface of the patient's hand (without the fingers) is approximately 1% of their body surface over all age groups

Burn wound depth

First degree: Red, dry and painful and are often deeper than they appear, sloughing the next day

Second degree: Red, wet and very painful. There is an enormous variability in their depth, ability to heal, and propensity to hypertrophic scar formation

Third degree: Leathery in consistency, dry, insensate, and waxy. These wounds will not heal

Fourth degree: Involve underlying subcutaneous tissue, tendon, or bone

Circumferential components

To allow for monitoring and prompt decompression if needed

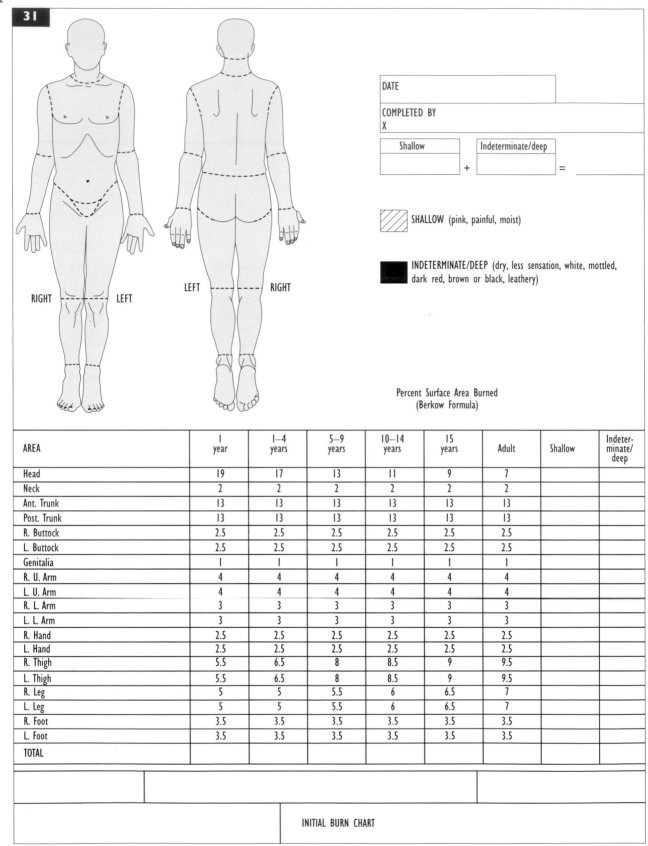

31

DATE

COMPLETED BY
X

Shallow		Indeterminate/deep		
	+		=	

///// SHALLOW (pink, painful, moist)

■ INDETERMINATE/DEEP (dry, less sensation, white, mottled, dark red, brown or black, leathery)

RIGHT — LEFT

LEFT — RIGHT

Percent Surface Area Burned
(Berkow Formula)

AREA	1 year	1—4 years	5—9 years	10—14 years	15 years	Adult	Shallow	Indeter-minate/deep
Head	19	17	13	11	9	7		
Neck	2	2	2	2	2	2		
Ant. Trunk	13	13	13	13	13	13		
Post. Trunk	13	13	13	13	13	13		
R. Buttock	2.5	2.5	2.5	2.5	2.5	2.5		
L. Buttock	2.5	2.5	2.5	2.5	2.5	2.5		
Genitalia	1	1	1	1	1	1		
R. U. Arm	4	4	4	4	4	4		
L. U. Arm	4	4	4	4	4	4		
R. L. Arm	3	3	3	3	3	3		
L. L. Arm	3	3	3	3	3	3		
R. Hand	2.5	2.5	2.5	2.5	2.5	2.5		
L. Hand	2.5	2.5	2.5	2.5	2.5	2.5		
R. Thigh	5.5	6.5	8	8.5	9	9.5		
L. Thigh	5.5	6.5	8	8.5	9	9.5		
R. Leg	5	5	5.5	6	6.5	7		
L. Leg	5	5	5.5	6	6.5	7		
R. Foot	3.5	3.5	3.5	3.5	3.5	3.5		
L. Foot	3.5	3.5	3.5	3.5	3.5	3.5		
TOTAL								

INITIAL BURN CHART

31 Burn extent is best estimated using a Lund–Browder chart that compensates for changes in body proportions with age.

Burn extent is best estimated using a chart that compensates for changes in body proportions with age (**31**). An expedient alternative is the Rule-of-Nines (**32**), in which the head and neck account for 9% of the body surface, each lower extremity accounts for 18%, each upper extremity accounts for 9%, and the anterior and posterior torso each account for 18% of the total body surface. For infants and young children, the Rule-of-Nines should be modified such that the head and neck are 18%, each lower extremity is 14%, each upper extremity is 9%, and the anterior and posterior torso are 18% each of the total body surface. For scattered or irregular burns, the entire palmar surface of the patient's hand represents approximately 1% of the body surface over all ages.

32 The Rule-of-Nines is an expedient method of estimating burn size, in which the head and neck account for 9% of the body surface, each lower extremity accounts for 18%, each upper extremity accounts for 9%, and the anterior and posterior torso each account for 18% of the total body surface. For infants and young children, the Rule-of-Nines has been modified such that the head and neck are 18%, each lower extremity is 14%, each upper extremity is 9%, and the anterior and posterior torso are 18% each of the total body surface. For scattered or irregular burns, the entire palmar surface of the patient's hand represents approximately 1% of the body surface.

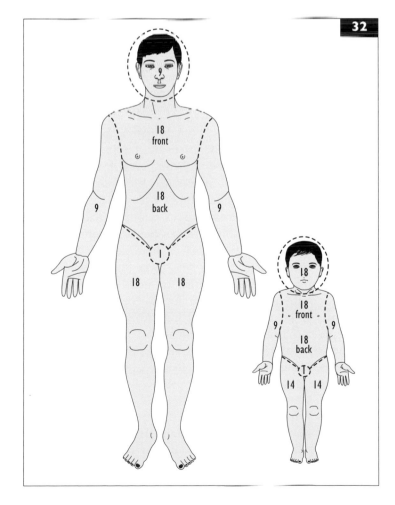

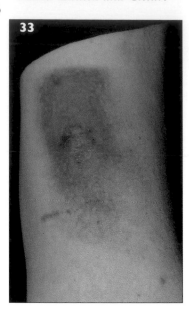

33 First-degree burns are red, dry and uncomfortable. They are often seen on the periphery of a second-degree burn.

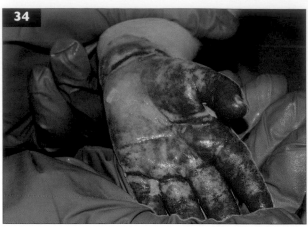

34 Second-degree burns are red, wet, and very painful. There is an enormous variability in their depth, ability to heal, and propensity to hypertrophic scar formation.

Burn depth is classified as first, second, third, or fourth degree (**33–36**). First-degree burns are red, dry, and uncomfortable and are often deeper than they appear, sloughing the next day. Second-degree burns tend to be moist and and very painful, but there is an enormous variability in their depth, ability to heal, and propensity to hypertrophic scar formation. Third-degree burns tend to be leathery, dry, insensate, and waxy. Fourth-degree burns involve underlying subcutaneous tissue, tendon, or bone. It can sometimes be difficult, even for an experienced examiner, to determine burn depth accurately on initial examination. As a general rule, burns are often underestimated in depth initially because there is commonly a microvascular thrombosis that occurs at the periphery of the wound that results in progressive tissue loss over the days following injury. Circumferential, or near circumferential, components should be noted because they represent areas where special monitoring, and sometimes escharotomy, are essential.

The initial estimate of burn size and depth is useful to help determine resuscitation fluid requirements. An accurate description of burn pattern is often an important aspect of later litigation. If the initial diagram is a quick middle-of-the-night estimate, it should be so stated on the diagram. If the initial estimate of depth is indeterminate, this can be so stated. This information is often documented in a burn diagram (**37**), which should be annotated as a working estimate unless very carefully done. In cases where litigation or charges may be expected, wounds ideally are photographed.

An accurate early determination of burn size, depth, and circumferential components impacts on resuscitation, transfer decisions, and prognosis. An accurate wound assessment is critical to operative planning. Accurate knowledge of burn depth, or actually the probability a wound will heal, is of enormous practical value. Many investigators have tried to develop tools to assist with the determination of a burn's propensity to heal, but there has been little practical success. For now, the eye of an experienced examiner remains the standard of burn evaluation and provides the most reliable basis for treatment planning.

DETERMINING THE TIME AND NEED FOR OPERATION

The primary issue that determines the need and timing of initial operation is the physiologic threat represented by the injury. In most patients, this is a function of injury size, although patients with small septic burns may also need prompt operation (**38, 39**). Many patients with small indeterminate depth injuries are best managed with an initial nonoperative approach while wounds evolve and depth becomes clearer. Generally, wounds that heal spontaneously in

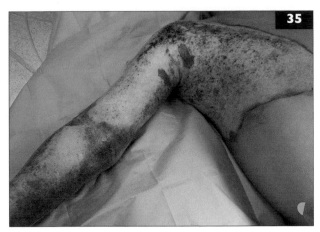

35 Third-degree burns are leathery, dry, insensate, and waxy. This wound demonstrates a peripheral second-degree component with central third-degree areas.

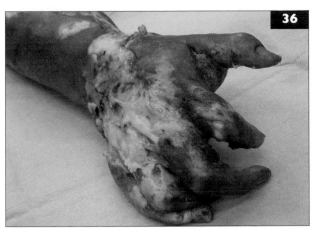

36 Fourth-degree burns involve underlying subcutaneous tissue, tendon, or bone.

37 A careful burn diagram should be completed at the time of initial evaluation. This should include an accurate representation of the wound size and pattern and a rough determination of wound depth. If the diagram is a working estimate, it should be so stated, as these diagrams can find their way into court months and years later.

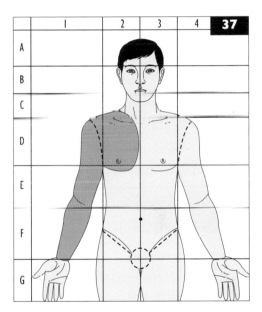

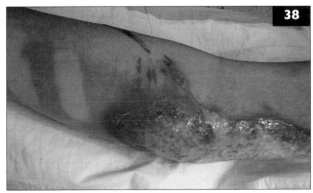

38 Patients with small septic wounds as pictured here may need prompt operation.

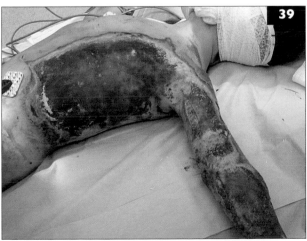

39 The physiologic threat posed by a larger burn is the most important consideration in operative timing.

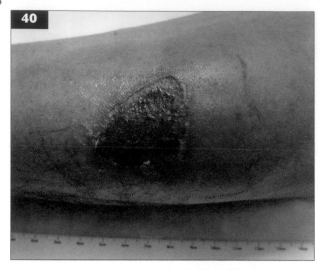

40 Patients whose burns are small but obviously full thickness at initial examination, such as many deep contact burns, are also usually better served by prompt operation as it truncates hospital stay.

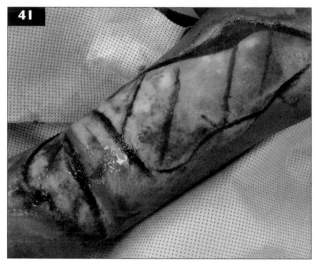

41 The objective of the initial operation is to identify, excise, and achieve biologic closure of all full-thickness components. Here, full-thickness components have been marked prior to beginning the excision. Operative time is decreased if these decisions are
not made in the midst of excision.

3 weeks or less are unlikely to become hypertrophic. It is therefore optimal if one can clearly identify and graft only those very deep dermal and full-thickness areas of the wound that one anticipates will take longer than this to heal. A common approach to those with small mixed-depth wounds, such as scalds, is to treat them with topical therapy for 3–5 days, to minimize desiccation and infection. During this period, wound depth becomes clear. Painful debridements are not practiced and much of this time can be spent in the out-patient setting. It is usually quite clear following this period which areas, if any, need to be excised and grafted and this is then performed. In this way, all grafts, donor sites, and second-degree burns are generally healed by 3 weeks. Patients whose burns are small but obviously full thickness at initial examination are also better served by prompt operation as it truncates hospital stay (**40**).

Patients with larger and deeper injuries, generally greater than 20% of the body surface, benefit from a more aggressive surgical approach, as the injury size alone presents a physiologic threat. These patients may do better if their full-thickness component is excised and closed during the first few days, prior to the development of wound colonization and systemic inflammation. The objective of the initial operation is to identify, excise, and achieve biologic closure of all full-thickness components (**41**). When the wounds are very large, generally greater than 40%, this may require staged procedures. If the wound involves more than 50% of the body surface, or if the patient is particularly fragile, temporary biologic closure can be achieved with human allograft, Integra®, or other temporary wound closure material. Wounds are later resurfaced with autograft when donor sites have healed. However, in most patients, immediate autografting is generally possible.

TECHNIQUES OF BURN WOUND EXCISION

Burn wounds are generally excised at one of five levels: (1) sharp debridement of loose devitalized tissue; (2) layered deep dermal excision; (3) layered excision to viable subcutaneous fat; (4) fascial excision; (5) subfascial excision of deep devitalized tissues. Wounds that are superficial and are clearly likely to heal require no excision and are simply cleansed and treated with topical medications or temporary biologic dressings. Some authors have advocated very superficial excisions of such wounds, feeling that removal of the thin amount of overlying eschar will facilitate more rapid healing, but there exist no compelling data to support this practice. Topical proteolytic enzymes may have a role in such injuries and have proven useful as an adjunct in some programs of care. They have not been widely adopted because current formulations either are too weak to be effective, or may damage underlying normal tissue. However, many programs use them quite successfully.

Layered excision to viable deep dermis is appropriate for those second-degree burns felt to be deep enough that spontaneous healing will be prolonged, i.e. greater than 3 weeks, with a resulting high incidence of hypertrophic scarring. This is especially true in areas where the skin is thin and has few appendages, such as the volar forearm. If too superficial a burn is managed in such a manner and an overlying sheet graft is placed, unsightly subgraft cyst formation can occur as remnant skin appendages

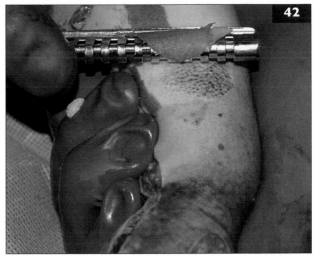

42 Layered excisions can be done with hand-held or powered dermatomes. Tourniquets or dilute epinephrine clysis will markedly reduce blood loss.

lose their natural drainage. Layered dermal excisions are generally only appropriate when it is clear that a result better than that obtainable with spontaneous healing will occur. The excisions can be done with hand-held or powered dermatomes (**42**). Excisions to this depth can be associated with substantial capillary bleeding, so it is important to use techniques to minimize blood loss (Textbox: Layered excision technique).

LAYERED EXCISION TECHNIQUE

Most burn excisions can be performed using a layered technique, preserving remnant viable subcutaneous fat and deep dermis. These excisions are more difficult than fascial excisions because tissue viability is hard to judge and bleeding can be impressive. They can be effectively and safely done over extensive areas using the following technique:
- Map the areas requiring excision with a surgical marker.
- Generously insufflate underlying tissue with dilute (0.5 µg/ml concentration) epinephrine solution, or exsanguinate an extremity and apply a proximal pneumatic or elastic tourniquet.
- Perform the marked excision briskly with hand-held or powered dermatome.
- Judge the adequacy (depth and breadth) of excision and modify if needed.
- Electrocoagulate larger bleeders and pack remaining wound in gauze moistened with dilute epinephrine solution, removing any proximal tourniquets.

Layered excision to viable subcutaneous fat is indicated particularly in smaller full-thickness burns to facilitate retention of a normal body contour. Capillary density in this wound is less than that of a deep dermal wound, much like cutting a forest horizontally at the level of the tree-trunks instead of the tree-tops. Therefore, graft 'take' here is less reliable, although generally limited more by inadequate excision of nonviable fat than it is by the lesser capillary density. These excisions can be performed with hand-held or powered dermatomes (Textbox: Layered excision technique). A pleasing cosmetic result generally occurs when sheet grafts are placed on viable subcutaneous fat. It is important to place the graft so that it will conform nicely to the many small irregularities in such a wound bed, and that no fat is left exposed, as this predictably leads to fat desiccation and graft loss. Widely meshed grafts do poorly on fat.

Fascial excisions are done infrequently, but are indicated if burns involve subcutaneous fat or in patients with massive, full-thickness burns in whom the risk of graft loss on extensive wounds excised to subcutaneous fat represents a threat to their life. These excisions are best performed with traction and coagulating electrocautery, a combination which provides excellent hemostasis and a well-defined wound bed that will reliably accept autograft (**43** and Textbox: Fascial excision technique). It is ideal to control the plume from the electrocautery unit, and

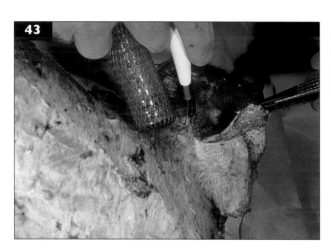

43 Fascial excisions are best performed with traction and coagulating electrocautery, a combination which provides excellent hemostasis and a well-defined wound bed that will reliably accept autograft.

FASCIAL EXCISION TECHNIQUE

Fascial excisions are infrequently required, being appropriate in larger and much deeper injuries. They can also be associated with substantial bleeding, but can be safely and effectively performed using the following technique:

- Clearly plan the excision to be done, marking those areas that must go to fascia.
- Incise the entire margin, through eschar, with coagulating electrocautery. The plume can be controlled with a high-efficiency suction device.
- With firm traction applied counter to excision, divide fibroareolar tissue and vessels at suprafascial level with coagulating electrocautery.
- Judge the adequacy (depth and breadth) of excision and modify if needed. A marginal layered excision is often needed, and can be blended to the fascial bed.
- Electrocoagulate larger bleeders and pack remaining wound in gauze moistened with dilute epinephrine solution.
- Marsupialization of wound edges with absorbable sutures, or tapering with layered excision, may help to de-emphasize contour deformaties.

this is effectively done with a high-efficiency suction device, many newer models having this as part of the electrocautery hand-piece.

Subfascial excisions, really excisional debridements of devitalized deep tissues, are required in high-voltage or, occasionally, in very deep thermal burns. Exploration of muscle compartments through standard fasciotomy incisions will allow significant areas of myonecrosis to be defined. Definitive closure of such wounds can be difficult. Vacuum assisted closure devices are useful to prepare such wounds for grafting. Occasionally local or distant flaps may be needed.

Attention, by both the surgeon and the anesthesiologist, to the physiologic status of the patient should be continuous and conscientious throughout the operation. Constant communication between teams will ensure physiologic stability, an absolute prerequisite for acute burn operations of the magnitude done today. Because of their absent epidermis and the frequent need for wide exposure, burn patients undergoing even simple operations are prone to hypothermia. This should be anticipated and prevented, as this will ensure optimal clotting and minimize physiologic stress. Although uncomfortable for operating room staff, this is best done with environmental heating.

pneumatic tourniquet and wrapping the extremity in a hemostatic dressing prior to tourniquet deflation; (3) executing all layered torso excisions after subeschar epinephrine clysis; (4) conducting all fascial excisions with traction and coagulating electrocautery; (5) performing major layered excisions as early as possible after injury prior to the development of wound hyperemia; and (6) strictly maintaining intraoperative normothermia. Layered excisions are performed using a variety of hand-held, gas powered, and electric dermatotomes of various sizes. Fascial excisions are best done combining traction with coagulating electrocautery. When using electrocautery, the plume can be controlled with a high-efficiency suction device. Ideally, burn operating rooms have highly efficient heating systems. To maintain normothermia for a widely exposed patient undergoing a large burn operation can require operating room temperatures of 90–100°F (~32–38°C) or higher. This may be uncomfortable for operating staff, but patients will tolerate extensive operations with greater stability, while maintaining innate clotting mechanisms.

TECHNIQUES TO MINIMIZE BLOOD LOSS

Published estimates of blood losses associated with acute burn operations are in the range of 3.5–5% of the blood volume for every 1% of the body surface excised. The primary reason for these large losses relates to the use of bleeding as an endpoint for excision. Free capillary bleeding informs the surgeon that the tissue is viable. However, there are other equally accurate methods of determining viability on inspection. Moist yellow fat, patent small blood vessels, the absence of thrombosis of small vessels, and the absence of extravascular hemoglobin are all consistent with viable tissue in a dry field. Reliable identification of the viability of excised wounds that are not bleeding is an acquired skill. It must be self-taught or learned. It is an essential skill that may be difficult to master or maintain if one is not doing these procedures frequently (**44**).

Several methods in combination will markedly reduce intraoperative bleeding: (1) clearly planning the excision to be performed prior to beginning; (2) performing all extremity excisions after inflation of a

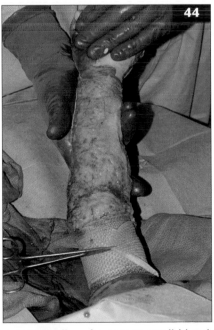

44 Bright, moist yellow fat, patent small blood vessels, the absence of thrombosis of small vessels, and the absence of extravascular hemoglobin are all consistent with viable tissue in a dry field. Note the presence of a proximal tourniquet.

GRAFT FIXATION AND POSTOPERATIVE WOUND CARE

Time spent securing grafts carefully in the operating room is time very well spent. Graft fixation techniques must: (1) eliminate shear between grafted surfaces and overlying grafts; (2) prevent desiccation and colonization of open interstices in meshed grafts; and (3) diminish hematoma and serous collection beneath sheet grafts. Proper attention to postoperative dressings will minimize the degree to which the patient must be immobilized to protect the integrity of fresh grafts, allowing physical therapy and rehabilitation efforts to proceed. Simple, but very carefully applied gauze wraps work well on extremities. Tightly stretched mesh dressings can be secured over anterior torso grafts giving excellent fixation (**45**). Posterior torso grafts can be held stable with multi-layer layered gauze secured to the underlying soft tissues (**46**). Standard tie-over dressings are useful for small grafts in many locations (**47, 48**). It is ideal to minimize the use of staples and sutures, as they must be subsequently removed. It is the dressings that hold the grafts in position after surgery, not staples or sutures. Carefully applied dressings and selective use of tissue glues are excellent substitutes.

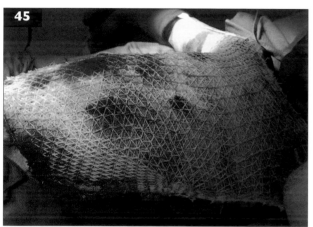

45 Tightly stretched mesh dressings can be secured over anterior torso grafts giving excellent fixation. The gauze mesh is here secured with staples. Subsequent traction on the gauze presents the staples for removal, so retained staples are infrequent.

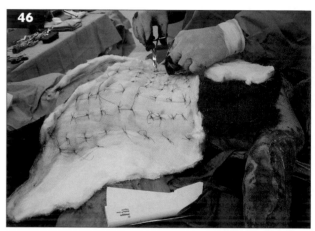

46 Posterior torso grafts can be held stable with multi-layer layered gauze secured to the underlying soft tissues.

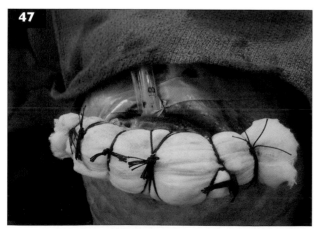

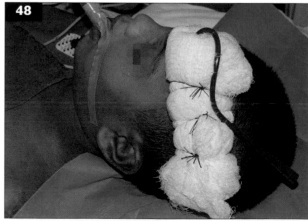

47, 48 Standard tie-over dressings are useful for small grafts in many locations. They can be dry (**47**) or wet with antiseptic solutions, sometimes via imbedded catheter (**48**).

Table 11 Characteristics of an idealized skin substitute

- Inexpensive
- Has a long shelf life without refrigeration
- May be used off-the-shelf on any patient
- Nonantigenic, nonallergenic
- Durable and easy to work with mechanically
- Flexible and contours to irregular surfaces well
- Physiologic vapor barrier
- Excellent bacterial barrier
- Easy to secure in position
- Vascularizes rapidly
- Grows with a child
- Can be applied in one operation
- Does not become hypertrophic
- Does not need surfacing with split-thickness autograft

Table 12 Principal characteristics of available temporary skin substitutes

Porcine Xenograft (Brennan Medical, St. Paul, MN):
- Adheres to coagulum
- Provides excellent pain control

Biobrane (Dow-Hickham, Sugarland, TX):
- Bilaminate
- Fibrovascular in-growth into inner layer

Acticoat (Smith & Nephew, Hull, UK):
- Nonadherent
- Delivers low concentration of silver

Aquacel-Ag (Convatec, Princeton, NJ):
- Absorptive hydrofiber
- Delivers low concentration of silver

Split-thickness allograft:
- Vascularizes
- Provides durable temporary closure

Various semipermeable membranes:
- Provide vapor and bacterial barrier

Various hydrocolloid dressings:
- Provide vapor and bacterial barrier
- Absorb exudate

Various impregnated gauzes:
- Provide vapor and bacterial barrier
- Allow drainage

Glycerol-preserved allograft (Euro Skin Bank, NL)

SKIN SUBSTITUTES

There is no currently available, widely useful, permanent skin substitute. Skin substitutes play an important supporting role in burn care, but currently, that is the extent of their utility. Most burns in most patients are optimally closed with split-thickness autograft. Someday, we will have available a practical skin substitute (*Table 11*). When available, a practical definitive skin substitute will have an enormous impact on the care of acute and reconstructive burn patients. From a practical perspective, skin substitutes now available play an adjunctive role only and are designed to be either temporary or permanent.

Temporary skin substitutes (*Table 12*), or biologic dressings, provide protection from mechanical trauma, a physiologic vapor barrier, and a physical barrier to bacteria. They foster a moist wound environment with a low bacterial density that facilitates optimal wound healing, and are most commonly used in one of the following settings: (1) as a dressing on donor sites to facilitate pain control and epithelialization from underlying skin appendages; (2) as a dressing on clean superficial wounds to a similar end; (3) to provide temporary physiologic closure of deep dermal and full-thickness wounds after excision while awaiting autograft availability or patient stability; (4) as an overgraft above widely meshed autografts to prevent dessication or colonization of exposed interstices (**49**); (5) as a test graft in questionable wound beds.

Permanent skin substitutes provide multiple components of skin function, particularly protection from mechanical trauma, a physiologic vapor barrier, and a physical barrier to bacteria (*Table 13*). Components are designed to be permanently incorporated in grafted wounds (**50–52**). Currently available permanent substitutes provide only a portion of the function of skin: either epidermal or dermal replacement products are currently available. Hopefully a reliable autologous composite product will become widely available in the next decade, until then no skin substitute is as reliable as split-thickness autograft, which remains the standard of care (**53**).

Table 13 Permanent skin substitutes

Integra (Integra LifeSciences Corporation Plainsboro, NJ):
- Provides scaffold for neodermis
- Requires delayed thin autografting
- Expensive

AlloDerm (LifeCell, The Woodlands, TX):
- Cell-free human dermal scaffold
- Requires immediate thin autograft
- Expensive

Epicel (Genzyme, Cambridge, MA):
- Autologous epithelial sheets
- Fragile
- Expensive

Split-thickness allograft:
- Dermal component vascularizes
- Dermal component may be left beneath autograft

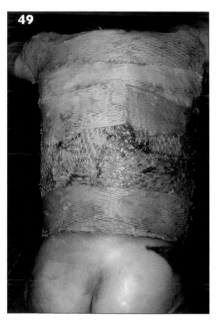

49 Meshed unexpanded allograft can be used to overgraft widely meshed autograft, protecting exposed interstices until epithelialized, at which time the allograft will slough.

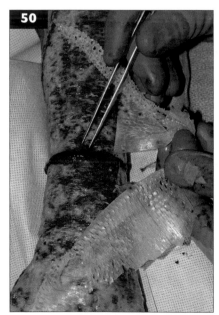

50 Integra (Integra LifeSciences Corporation Plainsboro, NJ) consists of an inner porous collagen and chondroitin-containing layer, designed to be vascularized by the host. An outer silastic layer serves as a temporary barrier. As illustrated here, it is removed prior to autografting 2 weeks after placement.

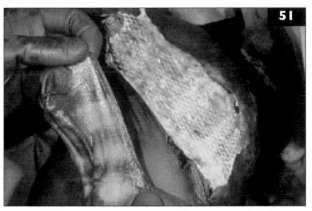

51 AlloDerm (LifeCell, The Woodlands, TX) is allogenic split-thickness dermis from which all cellular and antigenic elements have been removed. It is designed to be placed beneath a thin split-thickness autograft in one operation.

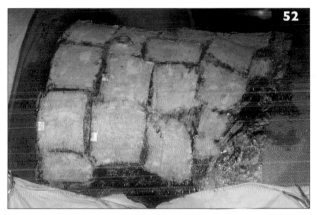

52 Epicel (Genzyme, Cambridge, MA).

53 No skin substitute is as reliable as split-thickness autograft, which remains the standard of care.

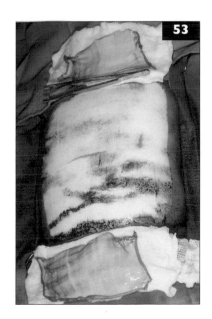

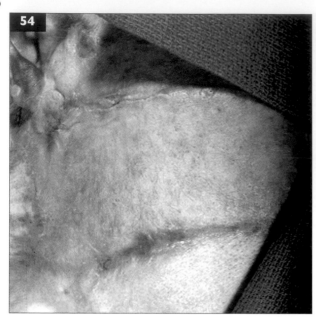

54 Over-deep scalp harvest can move hair onto the recipient site, an unsightly problem that can be managed to some extent with laser ablation of dark hair follicles.

DONOR SITE MANAGEMENT

There are a multitude of dressings that can be placed on donor sites, but most fit into one of two broad categories: (1) variations of open donor site care; (2) variations of closed donor site care. In the open group is any one of several nonocclusive dressings; in the closed category are all occlusive and hydrocolloid dressings. Open donor site management, using fine mesh gauze or vaseline impregnated dressings of various types or medicated ointments, is forgiving of donor site colonization and fluid collections. Their major disadvantage is the predictable discomfort that occurs over the first few days, until the dressing dries, forming a scab-like barrier over the wound. This pain can be minimized by injecting long-acting anesthetic agents, such as bupivacaine, beneath donor site wounds prior to emergence from anesthesia. The closed group of dressings include a wide variety of impermeable and semipermeable membranes and hydrocolloid dressings. The major advantage of this style of donor site management is the reduced pain associated with

their use. The major disadvantage of this group is their relative inability to tolerate fluid collections and wound colonization. When such occurs, they often need to be unroofed or removed, with a resulting donor site which can be more painful than it would have been had an open dressing been used from the outset. In posterior and large donor sites, open donor site management seems more practical, accepting the associated pain and medicating the patient appropriately. For small anterior donor sites, closed management works well in many patients. Any sutures used to secure donor site dressings are ideally placed within the area of the harvested epidermis so that no suture track epithelialization will occur with resulting unsightly suture track marks. When using the scalp as a donor, especially in young children, it is important not to harvest so thick that hair follicles are moved. This can result in alopecia at the donor site and unsightly hair growth at the recipient site (**54**). More recently, such morbidity can be managed to some extent with expanded flaps at the donor site and laser ablation of dark hair at the recipient site.

CASE PLANNING AND INTRAOPERATIVE POSITIONING

Speed is an excellent hemostatic agent. Operations should be conducted briskly after complete planning. Intraoperative position changes should be carefully planned. Many times, creative intraoperative positioning can obviate the need for position changes. Surgeons should know where they are operating and where available donor sites are. Positioning aids can be engineered into burn operating rooms, as should high-efficiency heating circuits. An inexpensive and highly effective positioning aid involves the use of an overhead suspension system (**55**).

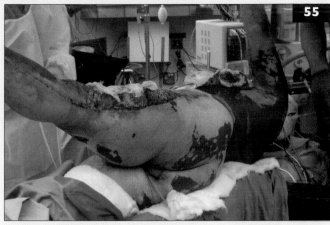

55 An overhead suspension system is an inexpensive and highly effective positioning aid for burn surgery.

AUSTERE ALTERNATIVES: INITIAL EXCISION AND CLOSURE

In many parts of the world, burn operating rooms are not heated, blood bank resources are limited, and perioperative intensive care is not an option. Planning burn excisions must acknowledge these realities. The aggressive early excisions performed in resource-rich units are simply not practical in many places. In this setting, burn wound sepsis is a common problem, and may be addressed by breaking total excision up into several procedures. Techniques to limit blood loss, such as dilute epinephrine clysis and tourniquets, are especially useful. Expensive topical agents, such as sulfamylon, are not available. Less expensive options, such as Dakin's solution, can be considered. Powered dermatomes and meshing devices are luxuries not often available. The Watson or Humby knife, often with resharpened blades, remains an important tool for excision and skin graft procurement (**56**). Expensive skin substitutes and temporary membranes are not usually available, so immediate autografting may be even more attractive. Excised wounds left open are generally better tolerated than unexcised wounds.

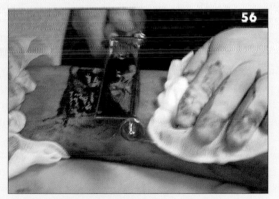

56 The aggressive early excisions performed in resource-rich units are simply not practical in many places. In many parts of the world, burn operating rooms are not heated, blood bank resources are limited, and perioperative intensive care is not an option. Planning burn excisions must acknowledge these realities. Free-hand blades remain important tools where powered devices are not available.

CHAPTER 6

RESPIRATORY ISSUES

'By failing to prepare, you are preparing to fail.'
Benjamin Franklin (1706–90),
printer, scientist, political appointee, author.

'Natural forces within us are the true healers of disease.'
Hippocrates (460–370 BCE), Greek physician.

INHALATION INJURY

Superheated air, products of combustion, hot liquid, or steam cause serious injury to the delicate tissues of the upper airway and lung. Clinical consequences include upper airway edema, bronchospasm, small airway occlusion, loss of ciliary clearance, increased dead space, intrapulmonary shunting, decreased lung and chest wall compliance, tracheobronchhitis, and pneumonia. Unfortunately, the degree to which these complications will develop is impossible to predict in individual patients. Even more problematic is that there are no specific therapies for inhalation injury. Our job is simply to provide general supportive care through observation and good pulmonary toilet, while managing complications if and when they arise.

The diagnosis of inhalation injury remains clinical, based on a history of closed space exposure, facial burns, burned nasal hairs, and carbonaceous debris in the mouth or sputum (**57**). Gas exchange and chest radiographs are usually normal for the first 2–5 days after injury, until slough of endobronchial debris occurs. Fiberoptic bronchoscopy may be used to support the diagnosis when it reveals carbonaceous debris, ulceration, or erythema, but cannot exclude inhalation injury in the setting of a very fine smoke that does not deposit in the upper airway (**58**). Technetium scanning has been used to confirm the clinical diagnosis, with injured parenchyma

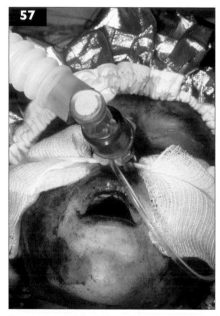

57 The diagnosis of inhalation injury remains clinical, based on a history of closed space exposure, facial burns, burned nasal hairs, and carbonaceous debris in the mouth or sputum. This child has the stigmata of inhalation injury.

demonstrating patchy clearance delay, but the technique has not been widely adopted and does not stratify severity.

The immediately life-threatening consequence of inhalation injury is upper airway edema. This results from direct thermal injury usually compounded by the diffuse capillary leak associated with a large surface burn. Hot liquid aspiration may cause catastrophic acute upper airway edema if it is not suspected and the airway promptly controlled (see **11**). Upper airway edema will have more immediate and catastrophic consequences in small children. Upper airway obstruction is heralded by hoarseness, retractions, and stridor, and should be followed by prompt endotracheal intubation (see Textbox: Endotracheal intubation and mechanical ventilation). Upper airway edema usually resolves in 2–3 days, and resolution can be facilitated by elevating the head of the bed and avoiding excessive fluid administration. Extubation can be considered when there is an airleak around the deflated cuff of an appropriately sized endotracheal tube at 20–30 cmH$_2$O, a level of consciousness consistent with airway protection, and acceptable gas exchange. In small children, a short course of steroids beginning 8–12 hr before extubation and continuing for a total of 24 hr may facilitate extubation without subsequent stridor. Bronchospasm can develop immediately after inhalation injury, especially in small children, but is usually responsive to inhaled beta-agonist agents.

Patients with inhalation injury usually have normal gas exchange for 48–72 hr after injury. Subsequently, endobronchial slough, small airway occlusion, and alveolar flooding occur. Compliance falls, gas exchange deteriorates, infection occurs, and respiratory failure develops. In the days preceding this predictable

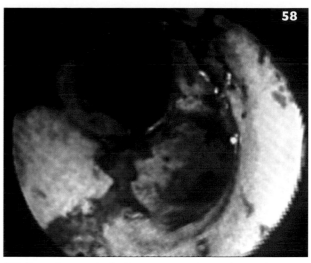

58 Bronchoscopic findings supporting a diagnosis of inhalation injury include carbonaceous debris, ulceration, or erythema.

deterioration, large excisions are well-tolerated, allowing providers to manage respiratory failure without worrying about simultaneous overwhelming wound sepsis. Most inhalation injury survivors have clinically normal long-term lung function.

ENDOTRACHEAL INTUBATION AND MECHANICAL VENTILATION

Endotracheal intubation and techniques of mechanical ventilation have salvaged many thousands of burn patients. Although it was not widely employed until the 1950s, the concept of endotracheal intubation and mechanical ventilation is ancient, probably dating back 500 years to Andreas Vesalius, who ventilated animals by breathing through an intratracheal reed passed through the neck. After the American Civil War, a multi-talented German surgeon, Friedrich Trendelenburg, did an operation while ventilating a patient via a tube passed through a temporary tracheotomy and British surgeon McEwen performed the first oral intubation for anesthesia. During this postwar era, George Poe, a Civil War veteran and manufacturer of the new anesthetic nitrous oxide, developed probably the first positive-pressure ventilator with the technical assistance of Arthur Ostrander, a small boy who helped him overcome his physical disabilities. During the First World War, British surgeons Magill and Macintosh developed much more effective techniques of oral and nasal endotracheal intubation. Intubating tools that bear their names are still in wide general use. Techniques of negative-pressure ventilation without an artificial airway became common during the polio epidemics of the 1940s, but were largely replaced by the combination of endotracheal intubation and positive-pressure ventilation after World War Two. The sophistication of current positive-pressure machines is remarkable.

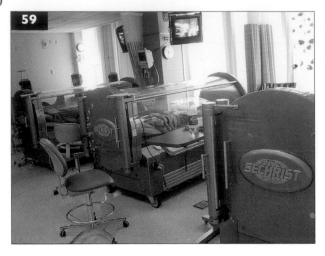

59 Hyperbaric oxygen treatments can be administered to patients requiring mechanical ventilation, but are not without risk and expense.

CARBON MONOXIDE AND CYANIDE EXPOSURES

Carbon monoxide (CO) is a colorless, odorless product of combustion that binds to heme-containing enzymes, including hemoglobin and mitochondrial cytochromes, interfering with oxygen transport and utilization, respectively. The standard of care for those exposed to carbon monoxide is 6 hr of 100% normobaric oxygen. In selected patients with more severe exposures, indicated by a carboxyhemoglobin level greater than 30% or neurologic changes, hyperbaric oxygen has been proposed to reduce further the incidence of long-term neurologic complications. Hyperbaric oxygen treatments are not without risk and expense and some studies question their efficacy (**59**). Relative contraindications to hyperbaric treatment include hemodynamic instability, fever (increases risk of seizure activity), and wheezing or air trapping (increases risk of pneumothorax and air embolism during decompression). In general, access to hyperbaric therapy does not justify transport of burned patients away from centers of burn care. If hyperbaric therapy is being considered, central venous catheters should be placed in the groins if possible to prevent treating a patient with an occult pneumothorax, and endotracheal tube cuffs should be filled with saline instead of air so that decreased cuff volumes with compression do not result in an air leak during treatment.

Hydrogen cyanide can be recovered from the smoke of many structural fires and is detectable in the blood of some patients with severe inhalation injury. However, it is rapidly metabolized in well-resuscitated patients. Specific treatment for cyanide exposures is not without risk and expense and is not part of standard care.

RESPIRATORY FAILURE

Respiratory failure is a common occurrence after serious burns. The cause of respiratory failure in this setting is often a combination of systemic and pulmonary infection, fluid overload, hypo-proteinemia, small airway occlusion, and alveolar flooding. Management involves providing support of gas exchange while identifying and correcting the underlying pathology. The high CO_2 production typical of hypermetabolic burn patients can complicate management of respiratory failure in this setting.

Pneumonia or tracheobronchitis occurs in over half of patients with inhalation injury, secondary to loss of the ciliary clearance mechanism, small airway occlusion, alveolar flooding, and translaryngeal intubation. Signs of pulmonary infection include fever and purulent sputum. Radiographic infiltrates or lobar consolidation suggest pneumonia. In the absence of clear radiographic changes, a diagnosis of tracheobronchitis may be made. Antibiotic therapy is directed by sputum gram stain and cultures. Neither bronchoalveolar lavage nor protected specimen brush specimens are routinely required for diagnosis and management. Antibiotic treatment should not be prolonged beyond a 7–10 day therapeutic course. Pulmonary toilet is especially important in these patients, as sloughed endobronchial debris is prominent, ciliary clearance is usually compromised, and coughing often absent. Blind suctioning supplemented with toilet bronchoscopy is an important component of therapy.

If compliance and gas exchange are near normal (typically patients intubated for airway protection) mechanical ventilation endpoints are normal blood gases. As respiratory failure develops, achieving normal blood gases will require the use of high concentrations of oxygen and inflating pressures. In this setting, after ensuring that there is no mechanically correctable problem (typically ventilator dyssynchrony from undersedation or impaired chest wall compliance from overlying eschar), the endpoints of oxygenation and ventilation should be reset to physiologically acceptable ventilation (any P_aCO_2 with a pH over 7.2) and acceptable oxygenation (any P_aO_2 consistent with an S_aO_2 over 90%). This approach, called permissive hypercapnia, is associated with excellent outcomes (*Table 14*). This strategy strives to avoid application of high, potentially injurious, inflating pressures and volumes. Permissive hypercapnia should be avoided if there is a coincident head injury, as it may cause increased cerebral blood flow.

CHRONIC AIRWAY MANAGEMENT

Some burned patients will require protracted intubation. Tracheostomy may reduce discomfort and enhance pulmonary toilet, while reducing the risk of unplanned extubation. However, indication and timing for tracheostomy in burned patients remain controversial. Young children, in whom the long-term risks of tracheostomy appear higher, may be better served by relatively prolonged oral intubation. Adults with thick secretions and anticipated protracted respiratory failure may be better served by early

---

Table 14 Management of progressive respiratory failure

Failing gas exchange in patients with inhalation injury and respiratory failure is best managed in a step-wise fashion

- Address bronchospasm with nebulized beta-agonist agents
- Address poor chest wall compliance secondary to overlying eschar with escharotomies
- Address endobronchial secretions with frequent suctioning and toilet bronchosocopy if needed
- Ensure ventilator synchrony with adequate opiate and benzodiazepine infusions. Neuromuscular blockade may be required on occasion
- Reset endpoint of ventilation to a physiologic pH (7.2 or more). Allow gradual-onset hypercapnia as long as there is no head injury
- Reset endpoint of oxygenation to an arterial saturation of at least 90%, typically associated with an arterial oxygen content of 60 torr or greater
- Optimize positive end-expiratory pressure (PEEP). This is usually done most practically by bedside trial
- Optimize peak inflating pressure. This is best done by using pressure control mode targeting a tidal volume of 6–7 ml/kg, as long as total inflating pressures (positive inspiratory pressure [PIP] + PEEP) can be kept under 40 cmH₂O. In some patients with compromised chest wall compliance from eschar, violating this pressure cap does not result in transpleural pressures in an injurious range
- In those few patients in whom these measures are not sufficient, consider the use of innovative adjuncts, such as inhaled nitric oxide or extracorporeal support

tracheostomy. Ideally neck edema has resolved before tracheostomy is performed and overlying neck burns have been grafted. There are no absolutes in this field, patient needs should be individualized. Recently, percutaneous tracheostomy has been done in burn patients with excellent results (**60**).

Unplanned extubation is a great hazard in burn patients with facial and upper airway edema (**61**). Planning will help successful management of this too-often catastrophic problem. Sudden deterioration of mechanically ventilated patients can result from ventilator dysschrony, mechanical failure of the ventilator, unplanned endotracheal tube displacement within or outside the airway, tube obstruction, or pneumothorax. A calm but rapid evaluation is then important (*Table 15*). Prevention is the best strategy. Patients are less likely to experience unplanned extubation if they are adequately sedated (lightly asleep but arousable) and the tube is well-secured. A tube-tie harness system works well (**61**). Comfortable prophylactic restraints for patient safety are entirely reasonable (**62**).

WEANING AND EXTUBATION

Intubated burn patients can be particularly difficult to wean from the ventilator. Patients intubated for 1–3 days for airway protection or perioperative support present straightforward weaning problems. A catabolic patient recovering from a large burn, respiratory failure, and pneumonia, who has been intubated for several weeks, and has ongoing pain presents much more difficult weaning problems. However, an organized approach will lead to a high degree of success (*Table 16*).

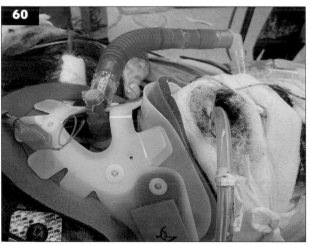

60 Percutaneous tracheotomy has been done in burn patients with excellent results.

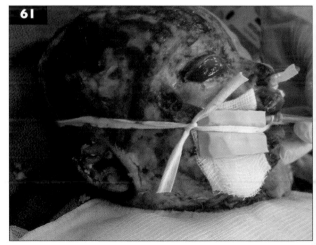

61 Prevention of unplanned extubation is the best strategy. A tube-tie harness system works well to secure the endotrachael tube. In this figure, the oral commisures have been protected with elastomer inserts.

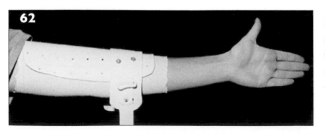

62 Comfortable prophylactic restraints for patient safety are entirely reasonable in intubated patients. In this figure, elbow immobilizers prevent inadvertent handling of the endotrachael tube and vascular access devices by the sedated patient.

Table 15 Rapid evaluation of deteriorating intubated burn patients

When there is a sudden deterioration of the intubated patient, there are five important possibilities to immediately consider: mechanical problem with the machine, tube obstruction, tube displacement out of the trachea, tube displacement into the right mainstem bronchus, or pneumothorax. Initial evaluation may be as follows:

- Disconnect the patient from ventilator and bag with a self-inflating bag (occluding the pop-off valve if necessary) at 100% F_iO_2. This eliminates and treats the possibility of mechanical problem with the system. If this is not the immediate solution:
- Bag ventilate the patient. If ventilations don't go in, you have an obstructed tube. Try to clear or suction the tube. If it cannot be quickly cleared, extubate, mask ventilate, and reintubate. If the tube was not occluded:
- Bag ventilate the patient. If the tube is not obstructed, you may have displacement out of the airway or down the right mainstem. If you hear gurgling in the hypopharynx, you probably have a tube displaced out of the airway or a cuff leak. If the former, extubate, mask ventilate, and reintubate. If the latter, inflate the cuff. If the tube seems to be in the airway:
- Bag ventilate the patient. Auscultate in the axillas. If the right-sided sounds are much louder than left-sided sounds you probably have a mainstem intubation. This can be confirmed by inspection of tube depth at the alveolar ridge (a properly sized and positioned tube should be 3×[tube size]cm from the alveolar ridge to the tip) or direct laryngoscopy showing a deep insertion (transverse mark below cords). Back the tube out cautiously and reassess. If neither of these is the cause:
- Bag ventilate the patient while auscultating both sides of the chest. Unilateral breath sounds are consistent with a pneumothorax. This can be tough to differentiate from a mainstem intubation in some situations, but is often accompanied by hemodynamic deterioration or hyperresonance. Inspection of the tube via direct laryngoscopy will reveal proper placement and depth of insertion. If you suspect a pneumothorax and don't have time for a chest X-ray, place a small catheter in the second interspace, mid-clavicular line, and later place a chest tube

The best management of unplanned extubation is prevention and preparation. Ensure good tube position and security on a regular basis. This is a most important vital sign

Table 16 Considerations for weaning and extubation of patients with serious burns

Seriously burned patients have extubation made more difficult by muscle catabolism, ongoing pain requiring medication, inhalation injury, reduced chest wall compliance, increased pulmonary secretions, and recovering pulmonary infection. Attention to the following points will enhance extubation success:

- Sensorium: the patient must be alert enough to guard their airway
- Airway patency: upper airway edema must be resolved to the degree that there is an audible airleak around a properly sized endotracheal tube ({16+[age in years]}/4) with cuff deflated at a moderate inflating pressure (approximately 20 cmH$_2$O). A 24-hr course of steroids (e.g. dexamethasone 0.5 mg/kg IV every 8 hr) may be useful in selected patients, particularly young children, to reduce airway edema
- Muscle strength: strength must be adequate for ventilation. An indirect measure of this is a tidal volume of 6–10 ml/kg with continuous positive airway pressure of 5 cmH$_2$O and a negative inspiratory force <-20 cmH$_2$O. A rapid, shallow breathing index (RR/TV) <105
- Pulmonary toilet: patients recovering from inhalation injury often have reduced ciliary clearance in the face of increased secretions from pneumonia and tracheobronchitis. They must be alert enough to cough and cooperate with suctioning. Frequent chest physiotherapy will help greatly with airway clearance
- Compliance: combined chest wall and lung compliance must be high enough that the work of spontaneous breathing is not excessive. Indirect measures of this are a measured static compliance of at least 50 ml/cmH$_2$O and tidal volumes of at least 10 ml/kg with moderate inflating pressures (<20 cmH$_2$O)
- Gas exchange: an intrapulmonary shunt <20%, indicated by a P_aO_2/F_iO_2 ratio greater than 200

The patient must be alert enough to guard their airway. Sedative medicines must usually be tapered prior to a planned extubation. Introduction of a short-acting sedative, such as Propofol or Dexmetomidine, 8–12 hr prior to a planned extubation allows longer-acting opiates and benzodiazepines to be more aggressively weaned prior to a planned extubation. Airway patency can generally be assumed to be adequate if facial swelling is resolved and there is an audible airleak around the deflated cuff of a properly sized endotrachael tube at an inflating pressure of 20 cmH$_2$O. Muscle strength must be adequate for ventilation. A spontaneous tidal volume of 6–10 ml/kg on continuous positive airway pressure of 5 cmH$_2$O and a negative inspiratory force less than 20 cmH$_2$O suggest adequate strength. Combined chest wall and lung compliance must be high enough that the work of unsupported breathing is not excessive. Indirect measures of this are a measured static compliance of at least 50 ml/cmH$_2$O and tidal volumes of at least 10 ml/kg with inflating pressures less than about 20 cmH$_2$O. An intrapulmonary shunt less than 20%, indicated by a P_aO_2/F_iO_2 ratio greater than 200, is desirable. A rapid shallow breathing index <105 may be predictive of successful extubition. After extubation, pulmonary toilet should be continued and patients closely monitored. Common reasons for extubation failure are progressive fatigue, lowered tidal volumes, atelectasis with shunting, and postextubation stridor. The latter is particularly common in young children. Such children usually do well if reintubated with a smaller tube, given 24 hr of intravenous steroids, and extubated again in 24 hr.

AUSTERE ALTERNATIVES

In austere environments respiratory support can be severely limited. In many locations, intubation and mechanical ventilation are simply not possible. In such circumstances, if burns are otherwise potentially survivable, elevation of the head and avoidance of fluid overload are especially important (**63**). The absence of intubation and mechanical ventilation may create a situation of *de facto* rationing when faced with large area burns. More difficult is when these resources are available but very limited. Again, careful forethought may help in rationing a limited resource wisely. Upper limits for injury severities that can be salvaged can be set in advance. Oftentimes, pediatric equipment is in more limited supply than adult equipment.

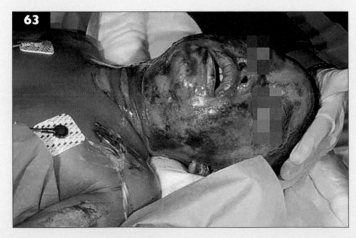

63 In some austere environments, intubation and mechanical ventilation are not possible. In such circumstances, if burns are otherwise potentially survivable, elevation of the head and avoidance of fluid overload are especially important.

CHAPTER 7

BURN CRITICAL CARE

'The wise man avoids evil by anticipating it.'
Publilius Syrus (circa 100 BCE),
Roman actor and author, a former slave.

'Never let the same dog bite you twice.'
Chuck Berry (1926–present),
American Rock & Roll musician.

Critical care is an absolute requirement to salvage patients with large burns. Optimally, an intensive care capability is an embedded component of any burn program. In the United States, this care has been generally under the direction of the surgeons providing overall patient care, although close affiliation with intensivists is a successful model elsewhere. In either case, seamless coordination of surgical and intensive care is essential. A systems approach to care with frequent reassessment, much like a pilot's check-list approach, will reduce errors and omissions (**64, 65** and *Table 17* [overleaf]). Some of the critical care issues unique to burn patients will be discussed here.

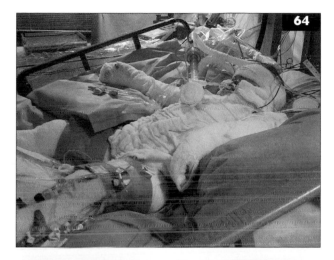

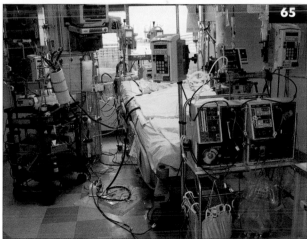

64, 65 The ICU is a complex environment making an organized approach essential. Protocol-driven care is extremely useful.

Table 17 Systematic approach to burn intensive care unit ward rounds
- Big picture
- Recent events
- Neurologic issues and plans
- Pain and anxiety issues and plans
- Hemodynamic issues and plans
- Pulmonary issues and plans
- Gastrointestinal issues and plans
- Nutrition issues and plans
- Infectious disease issues and plans
- HEENT issues and plans
- Genitourinary issues and plans
- Renal issues and plans
- Vascular access issues and plans
- Wound issues and plans
- Rehabilitation issues and plans
- Psychiatric issues and plans
- Family issues and plans
- Laboratory and X-ray issues and plans
- Care coordination and consultation issues and plans
- Other issues and plans
- Long-term care and follow-up issues and plans
- Documentation issues and plans

Table 18 An example of key objectives of a pain and anxiety management protocol

Ventilated acute:
- Tube security
- Covering background and procedural needs
- Opiate and benzodiazepine synergy
- Planning for extubation

Nonventilated acute:
- Avoidance of respiratory depression
- Covering background and procedural needs
- Opiate and benzodiazepine synergy

Chronic acute:
- Participation in rehabilitation efforts
- Covering background and procedural needs
- Perioperative comfort

Reconstructive:
- Perioperative comfort

NEUROLOGIC AND PAIN CONTROL ISSUES

Burn injury and its treatment are associated with significant pain and anxiety and assessment and management of this issue is an important component of daily care. A variety of age-appropriate assessment tools are available to facilitate monitoring. Regular documentation of these assessments will facilitate management. Ideally, a program-specific guideline is developed. A guideline that we have found to be very useful addresses four clinical states: mechanically ventilated acute patients, spontaneously breathing acute patients, acute patients during a protracted initial hospital course ('chronic acute'), and reconstructive patients. This protocol addresses background pain and anxiety, procedural pain and anxiety, and transition issues for each clinical state using a limited formulary and dose ranging (*Table 18*). Objective scoring is helpful. Pain and sedation scales, such as the Richmond Agitation Sedation Scale (RASS), can be used for tracking and titration of sedation. Particularly in older adults, ICU delirium can complicate care and can be tracked with tools such as the CAM-ICU. Opiate and benzodiazepine synergy are the cornerstone of effective pain and anxiety management, but adjunctive drugs, such as selected neuroleptics, are useful in particular patients. Nonpharmacologic tools can also be helpful in selected patients (**66**).

Peripheral neuropathies occur in about 5% of

patients with serious burns. These can be caused by direct thermal injury, direct nerve compression, or multiple metabolic derangements. Prompt decompression of tight ischemic extremities, attention to proper fitting of splints, careful intraoperative positioning, and close control of serum electrolytes may reduce the frequency of this complication (**67, 68**).

Cerebral edema and secondary seizures are associated with rapid development of hyponatremia, especially in small children. This can be avoided by minimizing the use of hypotonic fluid during resuscitation. Overly rapid correction of hyponatremeia has been associated with demyelination in the central nervous system. This can be minimized by close attention to serum electrolyte concentrations. Finally, patients with serious burns will often have episodes of decreased level of consciousness, if only secondary to pain and anxiety medications, particularly during interventions. If their original mechanism of injury was consistent with cerebral trauma or anoxia, liberal use of imaging is justified.

66 Opiate and benzodiazepine synergy are the cornerstone of effective pain and anxiety management, but nonpharmacologic tools are also very useful in selected patients. This photo illustrates music therapy as an adjunct during dressing change and wound cleaning.

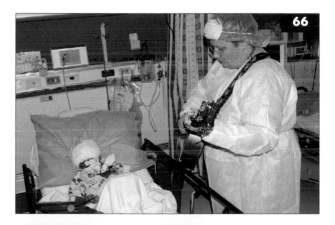

67, 68 Burn patients often require special positioning in the operating room or intensive care unit. Careful attention to pressure points or traction is important to minimize secondary peripheral nerve compression (**67**). Improper splint fit can also cause soft tissue injury (**68**).

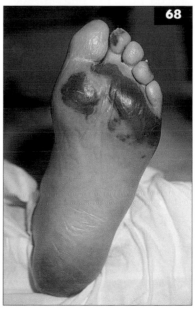

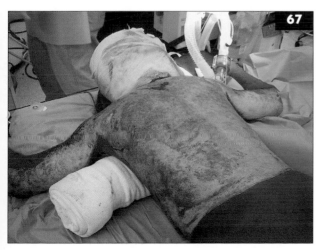

HEMODYNAMIC AND ELECTROLYTE ISSUES

A hyperdynamic circulatory and metabolic state predictably occurs in the days following a successful fluid resuscitation. This is characterized by a high cardiac output and low peripheral vascular resistance, temperature elevation, and increased metabolic rate. It is accompanied by worrisome muscle catabolism if adequate nutritional support is not provided (**69**). This physiology is driven by wound colonization, translocation of bacteria and their byproducts from the gut, and neurohormonal changes triggered by open wounds.

It can be difficult to determine the status of intravascular volume and fluid needs at this time. Episodes of sepsis are often preceded by recurrent capillary leak and increased fluid needs, further compounding the difficulty of determining intravascular fluid status. The best way to judge intravascular status and fluid needs is by a combination of careful serial physical examination, consideration of intravascular pressures, and selected laboratory data. Findings of particular importance include soft tissue edema, hepatic enlargement, central venous pressure, urine output, serum osmolality, and serum sodium concentration (**70**).

It is always important, particularly when managing children, to control the volume of fluid infusions, including all line flushes and medications into fluid calculations, to avoid inadvertent volume overload (**70**). If age-appropriate hemodynamic targets are not being met, the patient's hemodynamics should be evaluated and managed by optimizing, in order: preload, afterload, contractility, and heart rate. In most situations, hypoperfusion is related to inadequate preload, improved by administration of additional volume, or inadequate afterload, improved by cautious infusion of alpha-adrenergic or mixed alpha- and beta-adrenergic agents. Pure alpha-adrenergic agents should be used with caution, as they can be associated with splanchnic ischemia.

Serum electrolyte concentrations can take dangerous swings, particularly during the first days after resuscitation. Early on, electrolyte concentrations are strongly influenced by fluids infused for resuscitation, most patients developing an electrolyte profile similar to RL solution during resuscitation. Subsequently, transeschar flux of water has a major impact on these concentrations and should be anticipated. If nonaqueous topical medications are applied to wounds, free water loss assumes a prominent influence on serum electrolytes and free water should be administered. If aqueous topicals are used, transeschar leaching of sodium and potassium often occurs, requiring continued administration of isotonic crystalloid. As patients are fed, glucose enters the cells and is phosphorylated. This may contribute to the frequent occurrence of hypophosphatemia in the first days after serious

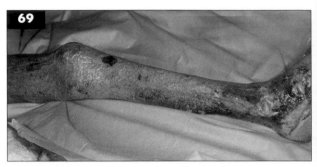

69 In the days following successful fluid resuscitation a hypermetabolic state develops. Nutritional support is essential to avoid the muscle catabolism demonstrated by this patient.

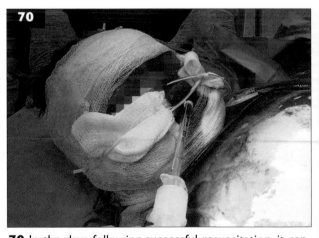

70 In the days following successful resuscitation, it can be difficult to determine the status of intravascular volume and fluid needs. Soft tissue edema and episodes of sepsis compound this. The best way to judge intravascular status and fluid needs is by a combination of careful serial physical examination, consideration of intravascular pressures, and selected laboratory data. This patient demonstrates significant post-resuscitation edema, but intravascular volume was normal by other measures. Regular physical assessment provides very useful information.

injury. Hypomagnesemia is common as well. Both can be problematic if not corrected. Rapid swings in serum electrolytes are associated with significant morbidity, so diligent electrolyte monitoring and replacement are critical components of care, particularly in the first days after resuscitation from a large injury.

Optimal management of predictable hypo-albuminemia remains controversial. After severe injury, hepatic albumin synthesis is reduced in favor of acute phase protein production. This reduced synthesis combined with enhanced albumin loss through open wounds causes sometimes profound hypoalbuminemia. How low one should allow serum albumin to fall has been an area of controversy for many years. In the postresuscitation period, it has been our practice to tolerate levels as low as 1.5 g/dl (15 g/l) as long as there is no enteral feeding intolerance, pulmonary dysfunction, or troublesome soft tissue edema. If serum albumin falls below 1.5 g/dl (15 g/l), or enteral feeding intolerance, pulmonary dysfunction, or troublesome edema develops, infusion of 1–2 g/kg/day of albumin (as 5% or 25% formulations) to a target of 2.0 g/dl (20 g/l) is justified. Current preparations are heat-treated and carry little risk.

VASCULAR ACCESS

Intraosseous lines can provide emergency access in children. Peripheral lines can provide temporary access for infusions. However, central venous access is required for most seriously burned patients throughout much of the acute hospitalization (Textbox: A severe attack of common sense). Properly functioning central lines provide access for infusion of fluid and medications and painless phlebotomy for laboratory tests. Central sites should be treated with great care if they are to last for the

A SEVERE ATTACK OF COMMON SENSE

In the early years of modern burn care, peripheral venous lines, placed by cutdown or percutaneously, were relied upon for chronic vascular access. Septic peripheral thrombophlebitis was common during those decades. In the 1980s, these methods were largely replaced by percutaneous central venous access using large steel needles through which single-lumen polyvinyl chloride lines were passed. Although incredibly useful, this technique had a high rate of bleeding and mechanical complications. In the late 1940s, a Swedish radiology and angiography trainee (who came from a family of fine watchmakers) at the prestigious Karolinska Institute, Dr. Sven-Ivar Seldinger (1921–1998), was trying to improve his technique of percutaneous cannulation when he had a self-described '*severe attack of common sense*'. He later recollected, '*I found myself with three objects in my hand – a needle, a wire, and a catheter – and in a split second I realized in what sequence I should use them: needle in, wire in, needle off, catheter on wire, catheter in, catheter advance, wire off.*' Dr. Seldinger first published his technique in 1953, and it gradually gained acceptance in angiographic circles, particularly after a 1966 publication that reported its use in cholangiography (and served as his doctoral thesis). It was not until the 1990s that it was widely adopted for vascular cannulation in the intensive care environment (the author of this monograph trained in surgery in the 1980s using exclusively through-the-steel needle cannulation). Seldinger's technique is now the standard of care for central cannulation and has protected thousands of patients from mechanical vascular access complications. Dr. Seldinger left academia at the height of his fame in 1967 to run the radiology department in the local hospital of his home city, Mora. Perhaps he has a lesson for us here as well.

duration of the hospitalization (and beyond) and if life- and limb-threatening complications (reported to occur in 4% of insertions) are to be minimized. Central veins are limited and will clot if cannulated with large catheters or clumsy technique. The incidence of thrombosis of these valuable sites may be reduced by using the smallest diameter catheter with the fewest number of lumens that will reasonably meet the patient's needs. Placement of central venous catheters, especially in small children, is an important skill to cultivate (*Table 19*).

Burn patients have frequent occult bacteremias with wound manipulation which may seed intravascular catheters, explaining a higher risk of catheter sepsis in this population. Periodic catheter site rotation is felt to decrease this incidence of catheter sepsis, although the issue remains controversial and specific practices vary. We are convinced that weekly rotation of catheters is a reasonable approach that minimizes both catheter-related sepsis and the mechanical complications associated with line insertion (**71**). This presumes that insertions are done carefully. Antiseptic catheters

may reduce the incidence of line sepsis, but there are no data that provide adequate evidence to indicate the need for change in line rotation policies in burn patients at the present time.

Arterial lines are useful in selected patients with respiratory failure who need frequent arterial blood gas monitoring or hemodynamically labile patients who require frequent blood pressure monitoring. Patients intubated for airway protection are well-managed with a pulse oximeter to monitor arterial oxygen saturation and an extremity cuff to measure blood pressure. Arterial lines infrequently become infected, probably because of the high blood flow rates, so they are only replaced if they malfunction, if the site becomes inflamed, or infection is suspected. Favored sites are dorsalis pedis and radial arteries. Femoral arterial lines can be safely inserted, but careful technique is required to avoid hemorrhage or distal ischemia. Brachial and axillary arterial lines should only be used with extreme caution because of the risk of ischemia to the hand in the former, and of cerebral embolization with vigorous flushing in the latter.

Table 19 Selected technical highlights of successful central venous cannulation

- Ensure proper sedation, appropriate lighting, sterile technique, adequate drapes, comfortable operator and patient positioning, and ready access to needed supplies before commencing insertion
- When placing upper body catheters, the patient is placed in Trendelenburg position, arms by the side, head slightly extended and turned to the contralateral side, the shoulders gently extended by a vertical towel roll between the scapulae. Extremes of position are avoided
- When placing upper body catheters, the catheter tip should reside in the superior vena cava, not the right atrium. This is facilitated by estimating the required intravascular length before insertion (the tip should be at about the sternomanubrial junction)
- Choose a catheter length that will not require substantial catheter length outside the venepuncture site. This is a more secure catheter
- It is not necessary to pass the full length of the dilator around the curves of the great veins, risking their injury. It is only necessary to dilate the overlying clavipectoral, cervical, or femoral fascia
- There is no place for force when placing central venous catheters. Forceful technique will never lead to successful cannulation, it will only lead to trouble
- When placing central venous catheters in the femoral position, puncture the skin well below the inguinal ligament and aim to puncture the vein in the femoral triangle, before the vein dives into the pelvis. In this location any vascular injury will be readily detected by obvious hematoma and pressure can be effectively applied. High puncture risks anterior wall laceration and retroperitoneal hematoma
- When you are not certain if a wire is intravenous or intraarterial, place a small diameter catheter over the wire and transduce it to be sure that you have not cannulated the artery. A small catheter will be less likely to cause arterial injury than a dilator and full size catheter
- Do not guidewire change the only catheter of a patient on vasopressors

NUTRITIONAL SUPPORT

Burns is a severely catabolic illness that requires specific support. This hypermetabolic physiology is poorly understood, but is demonstrated by all mammalian species and therefore may have survival value in nature. The response includes fever, increased metabolic rate, increased minute ventilation, increased cardiac output, decreased afterload, increased gluconeogenesis, insulin resistance, and increased skeletal and visceral muscle catabolism. Patients remain hypermetabolic until wound closure is complete and for a variable period thereafter. Accurate support of this physiology is essential. Overfeeding causes fatty infiltration of the liver, which can lead to hepatic dysfunction, and increased CO_2 production, which can exacerbate respiratory failure. Underfeeding causes muscle wasting and interferes with wound healing (**72**).

Nutritional support is ideally provided enterally, with tube feedings beginning during resuscitation. In patients with serious burns, the author's practice has been to begin intragastric tube feedings via a sump tube during resuscitation at about 10% of goal rate, monitoring intragastric residuals, abdominal distension, and bowel sounds. Many authorities consider postpyloric feedings to have substantial advantages, although monitoring of tolerance can be a bit more difficult. Tube feedings are gradually increased to a goal rate, based on formula, over the next 48 hr if aspirates remain less than twice an hourly rate and abdominal distension does not develop. Enteral feeding is preferred over parenteral feeding because this route better supports the gut barrier, may decrease bacterial translocation, is cheaper, and has fewer potential metabolic complications. As tolerance is established, nasogastric sump tubes are changed to soft feeding tubes, allowing distal migration. Some patients, especially those with large burns during the early resuscitation period or those with sepsis, do not tolerate enteral feedings at goal rates and supplemental parenteral nutrition, in addition to enteral feedings at low rates, is justified and generally very well and safely tolerated.

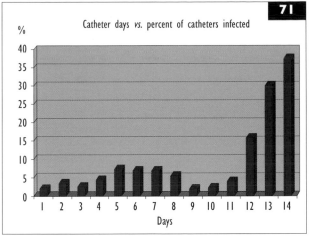

71 Weekly rotation of catheters is a reasonable approach that minimizes both catheter-related sepsis and the mechanical complications associated with line insertion. This figure reflects data collected on 1000 consecutive pediatric central venous catheters. Those dwelling more than 10 days had a much higher incidence of infection.

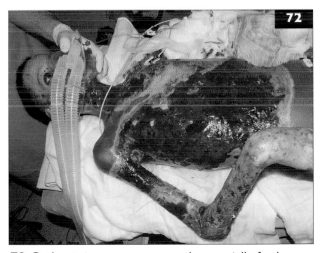

72 Cachexia is a very severe and potentially fatal complication of poor nutritional support in catabolic burn patients. This should be watched for by regular physical examination and weighing, sometimes supplemented by laboratory tests and indirect calorimetry.

Nutritional support must be individualized, just like fluid resuscitation. A rough initial estimate of energy needs in most patients is 25–35 kcal/kg/day; this can be refined with more accurate calculations, such as the Harris–Benedict equation (*Table 20*). Laboratory tests, such as albumin, prealbumin, and retinal binding protein can supplement bedside examination. Expired gas indirect calorimetry can also be useful as an adjunct to clinical monitoring. Resting energy expenditure can be roughly measured via indirect calorimetry. Multiplying resting energy expenditure by a factor of 1.5–1.7 provides an estimate of total energy expenditure and a nonprotein caloric target. Directed physical examination and weight, sometimes supplemented by indirect calorimetry or formula calculations, can be performed twice weekly to monitor the adequacy of nutritional support, much as one would monitor fluid infusions based on urine output.

Empirically, patients with large wounds to heal seem to do so more reliably when provided with large amounts of protein. A common target is 1.5–2.5 g/kg/day, which is well in excess of the needs of uninjured persons. Ideally, protein is not figured into caloric loads, which are provided as carbohydrate and fat.

An increasing body of literature suggests that control of hyperglycemia, generally via intravenous insulin, reduces the incidence of infection and fosters an anabolic state. How tightly to control serum glucose remains debated, as too tight control increases the risk of hypoglycemic episodes. Moderate control (target 110–150 mg/dl [1000–1500 mg/l]) via a well-monitored insulin infusion (serum glucose checked every 1–2 hr while on insulin infusions) has proven safe and effective.

Anabolic agents, such as recombinant human growth hormone, anabolic steroids, beta-agonists, and insulin-like growth factor have been used to accelerate donor site healing and restore earlier positive nitrogen balance. These agents may play an important role in burn care, but currently are not part of the standard of care. In most burn programs the use of anabolic agents, most commonly the anabolic steroid oxandrolone, is reserved for individuals with compromised healing or established nutritional deficiency. The use of such agents is expanding

COMPLICATIONS AND SEPSIS

Patients with serious burns are immunosuppressed. They have absent epithelial barriers and multiple invasive devices. They are subject to a number of septic complications until all of their wounds are closed. A deteriorating burn patient should be assumed to have a septic complication until proven otherwise. Burn patients, particularly those transferred between units, may harbor resistant organisms (**73**). Infection control measures should be rigorously followed to prevent cross infection. Many times, successful burn care requires management of a series of complications while pushing ahead with wound closure (*Table 21*). Constant vigilance on the part of providers facilitates early detection and effective treatment.

Table 20 The Harris–Benedict Equation provides an estimate of basal metabolic rate (BMR)

Calculated BMR can be multiplied by an injury or activity factor (commonly in burns from 1.5–1.7) to provide an estimate of caloric needs

BMR formula (traditional units)
Women: BMR = 655 + (4.35 × weight in pounds) +
  (4.7 × height in inches) - (4.7 × age in years)
Men: BMR = 66 + (6.23 × weight in pounds) +
  (12.7 × height in inches) - (6.8 × age in years)
BMR formula (metric units)
Women: BMR = 655 + (9.6 × weight in kilos) +
  (1.8 × height in cm) - (4.7 × age in years)
Men: BMR = 66 + (13.7 × weight in kilos) +
  (5 × height in cm) - (6.8 × age in years)

73

Pseudomonas aeruginosa	
AMPICILLIN	resistant
BACTRIM	resistant
CEFOTAXIME	resistant
CEFAZOLIN	resistant
CHLOROMYCETIN	resistant
AMIKACEN	resistant
GENTAMICIN	resistant
IMIPENEM	resistant
PIPERCILLIN	resistant
TOBRAMYCIN	resistant
CEFTAZIDINE	resistant
ACARCILLIN	resistant

73 Burn patients, particularly those transferred between units, may harbor resistant organisms. This resistance profile is not fictitious. Universal precautions and infection control policies should be rigidly followed to prevent cross-colonization with these difficult organisms.

Table 21 Common complications seen in patients with serious burns

Neurologic
- Transient delirium: occurs in up to 30% of patients. It usually resolves with supportive therapy. Anoxia, metabolic disturbance, and structural lesions should be considered
- Seizures: can complicate hyponatremia with cerebral edema or abrupt benzodiazepine withdrawal
- Peripheral nerve injuries: can occur from direct thermal injury or compression from compartment syndrome, constricting eschar, or tight splints in sedated patients
- Delayed peripheral nerve and spinal cord deficits can develop weeks after high-voltage injury secondary to small vessel thrombosis or demyelination

Psychiatric
- Post-traumatic stress disorder: occurs in up to 30% of burn patients. It can be exacerbated by inadequate pain and anxiety management

Cardiovascular
- Endocarditis: presents with fever and recurrent bacteremia, sometimes accompanied by a new murmur
- Suppurative thrombophlebitis: presents with fever and bacteremia, often without signs of local infection. Diagnosis may require ultrasonography or exploration of prior peripheral intravenous sites or cutdowns
- Hypertension: may occur most commonly in preadolescent boys and is best managed with beta-adrenergic blockers, once adequate pain and anxiety management are ensured
- Venous thromboembolic complications: are infrequent in young children. They are common enough in postpubertal and adult patients to justify prophylaxis. Careful venous cannulation and use of the smallest catheter that can meet the patient's needs will further reduce this complication
- Central venous and arterial catheter insertion complications: can be minimized by meticulous technique

Pulmonary
- Carbon monoxide intoxication: is managed with effective ventilation with 100% oxygen for 6 hr. Hyperbaric oxygen treatment is appropriate in selected patients with very severe exposure
- Pneumonia: may occur with or without inhalation injury and is treated with pulmonary toilet and antibiotics
- Respiratory failure: may occur early postinjury secondary to inhalation injury or late secondary to sepsis or pneumonia

Hematologic
- Neutropenia and thrombocytopenia: accompany sepsis and should trigger investigation for infectious complications
- Disseminated intravascular coagulation: is commonly secondary to sepsis and should prompt empiric treatment and search for septic foci
- Immunologic deficits: are common in serious burns. Prompt wound closure is the best treatment

Otolaryngologic
- Auricular chondritis: results from bacterial invasion of relatively avascular cartilage beneath ear burns, causing rapid destruction of the framework of the ear (**74**). It can be prevented by topical mafenide acetate
- Sinusitis and otitis media: can be caused by obstruction of the Eustachian tube by nasal endotracheal or gastric tubes. It is treated by relocation of tubes, antibiotics, topical decongestants, and occasional surgical drainage
- Complications of endotracheal intubation: include nasal alar and septal necrosis (**75**), vocal cord erosions and ulcerations, tracheal stenosis, and tracheoesophageal and tracheoinominate artery fistulae. The occurrence of such complications is minimized by proper tube position and size and attention to cuff pressures

(Continued overleaf)

74 Auricular chondritis can destroy the cartilaginous structure of the ear.

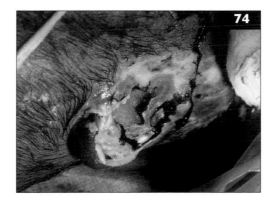

75 Endotracheal tube security is absolutely essential, but septal erosions should be avoided.

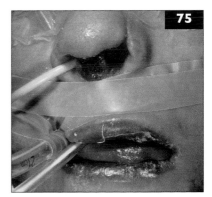

Table 21 Common complications seen in patients with serious burns (continued)

Enteric

- Hepatic dysfunction: can be secondary to splanchnic ischemia during resuscitation and presents as transaminase elevation. Late hepatic failure is usually secondary to sepsis and presents with elevated cholestatic chemistries and progressive synthetic failure
- Pancreatitis: can be secondary to splanchnic ischemia and begins with amylase and lipase elevation progressing through hemorrhagic pancreatitis
- Acalculus cholecystitis: can present as sepsis with rising cholestatic chemistries without localized signs in critically ill patients. Serial physical examination and ultrasound are generally diagnostic. Bedside percutaneous cholecystostomy is useful in unstable patients
- Gastric and duodenal ulcers: are caused by splanchnic ischemia during the early hours after injury. This can result in life-threatening bleeding or perforation. The risk is reduced by effective resuscitation and routine histamine receptor blockers and/or antacids
- Intestinal ischemia: is caused by splanchnic ischemia and can progress to infarction. It is prevented by effective resuscitation. It can occur later due to fulminating sepsis
- Small bowel overfeeding with perforation: can occur if postpyloric feeds are administered by pumps despite an unappreciated ileus. Prevention requires frequent abdominal examination
- *Clostridium difficile* colitis: presents with severe diarrhea and systemic toxicity. Burn patients exposed to antibiotics are at risk. Empiric treatment with enteral metronidazole or vacomycin is justified in toxic patients while awaiting titers

Ophthalmic

- Ectropia: caused by contractile forces of facial and eyelid burns; risks globe exposure and dessication. Tarsorrhaphy is infrequently helpful as contractile forces can cause these sutures to pull through the lids. Lid release is a more definitive and effective treatment (**76, 77**)
- Corneal ulceration: complicates corneal burns or corneal exposure and dessication. Superinfection can lead to corneal perforation and loss of vision (**78**). This dreaded complication can be minimized by vigilant globe lubrication and prompt correction of ectropia
- Symblepharon: are adhesions of the lid to the denuded conjunctiva following chemical burns or corneal epithelial defects complicating TEN. These can be minimized by daily examination and adhesion disruption (**79**)

Renal

- Early acute renal failure: follows inadequate perfusion during resuscitation, myoglobinuria, or abdominal compartment syndrome
- Late renal failure: complicates sepsis and multiorgan failure or the use of nephrotoxic agents

Endocrine

- Acute adrenal insufficiency: presents with variable degrees of hypotension, fever, hyponatremia, and hyperkalemia

Genitourinary

- Urinary tract infections: are common complications of bladder catheterization. They can be minimized by placing bladder catheters only when necessary
- Nephrolithiasis: is infrequent, but can be seen in immobilized burn patients. Typical pain, hematuria, or frequent infection should prompt investigation
- Candida cystitis: can be treated with antifungals administered systemically or by irrigation. If infections are recurrent, the upper tracts should be screened ultrasonographically

Musculoskeletal

- Exposed burned bone: may require complex flap closure. However, in most situations, debridement of exposed necrotic bone with a powered bit facilitates granulation tissue coming up through nutrient vessels, which supports subsequent autografting (**80**). Negative-pressure dressings seem to speed granulation in such settings
- Fractured and burned extremities: are best immobilized with external fixators while overlying burns are grafted (**81**). Burn patients with fractures in unburned extremities are often best managed with prompt internal fixation
- Heterotopic ossification: develops weeks after injury most commonly around deeply burned major joints such as the triceps tendon (**82**, *overleaf*). It presents with pain and decreased range of motion. Most patients respond to physical therapy, but some require excision of heterotopic bone to achieve full function
- Hypertrophic scar formation: is a major cause of long-term functional and cosmetic morbidity. It can cause deformity during protracted acute hospitalization and may require acute release to ensure optimal recovery (**83, 84**, *overleaf*). Later management tools include compression garments, massage, steroid injections, topical silicone, tuneable dye laser, Z-plasty, and incisional release surgery

76, 77 Lid release is the most effective and definitive treatment for eyelid ectropion.

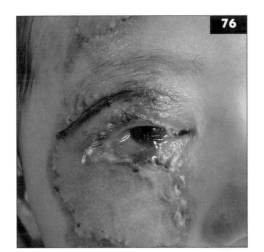

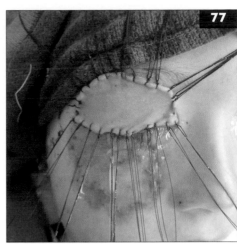

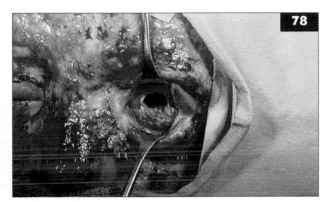

78 Infected corneal ulcers can lead to globe perforation, extrusion of the lens, and visual loss. Vigilant globe lubrication and prompt correction of ectropia will minimize the occurrence of this complication.

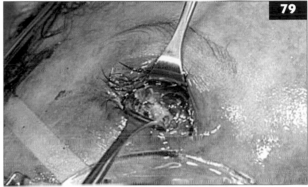

79 Symblepharon can be prevented by regular disruption of adhesions forming between a denuded globe and lid.

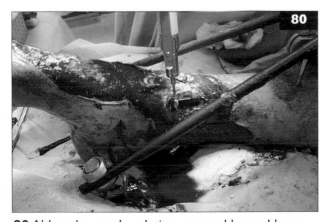

80 Although a crude solution, exposed burned bone is often best acutely managed by debridement of exposed necrotic bone with a powered bit, which facilitates granulation tissue coming up through nutrient vessels. Negative-pressure dressings seem to speed granulation in such settings.

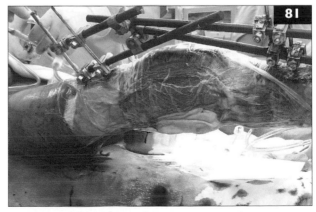

81 Fractured and burned extremities are best immobilized with external fixators while overlying burns are grafted. This extremity has an associated wound that is being treated with a negative-pressure dressing.

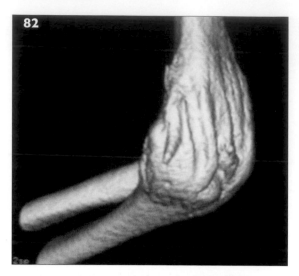

82 Heterotopic ossification develops weeks after injury most frequently around deeply burned major joints, most commonly at the elbow. As seen in this CT reconstruction, the bony excrescences may block elbow motion.

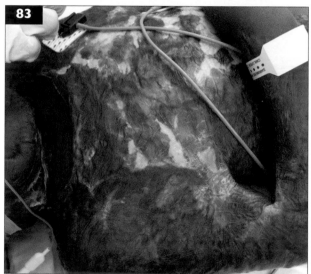

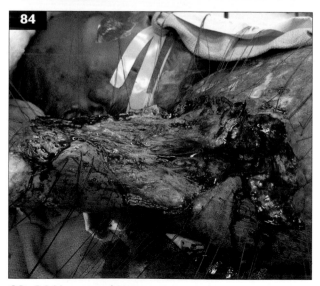

83, 84 Hypertrophic scar may require acute release to ensure optimal recovery at initial discharge.

Providers of burn care are frequently faced with febrile patients in whom sepsis is a worry, but not a certainty. Fever is a normal part of the hypermetabolic response. Most patients with significant burns are febrile, even when they are not septic. Overtreatment with broad-spectrum antibiotics is not in the best interest of individual patients. Prophylactic antibiotics do not seem to reduce the incidence of septic complications. How does one reconcile the fear of missed sepsis with the need to limit profligate antibiotic use? A common sense solution is first to do a physical exam, looking particularly at the wound, invasive devices, and recent surgical sites. If there is no apparent septic focus, patients can be divided into one of three categories: worrisome, intermediate, or not worrisome. Patients with coincident hypotension, lethargy, exacerbation of organ failures, extremely high temperatures, very high white blood cell counts, or plunging platelet counts are very worrisome. These patients can be cultured and placed on broad-spectrum antibiotics for 48–72 hours awaiting return of culture information. Patients who show none of these features are not worrisome and can be observed. The approach to those few who are intermediate between these categories must be individualized, with very fragile young or elderly patients perhaps given empiric antibiotics. The important point is that fever does not equate to infection, and fever should not result in automatic antibiotic administration. This practice fosters antibiotic resistance and is not in the patient's best interest.

Multiple organ dysfunction is a complication of shock-related tissue hypoxia and severe or repeated smaller infections. In burn patients, the sequence of events is commonly increasing obtundation, pro-

Table 22 Burn wound infections

Burn impetigo:
- loss of epithelium from previously epithelialized surface
- not related to local trauma

Burn-related surgical wound infection:
- infection in a surgically created wound which has not yet epithelialized
- includes loss of any overlying graft or membrane

Burn wound cellulitis:
- infection occurs in uninjured skin surrounding a wound
- signs of local infection progress beyond what is expected from burn-related inflammation

Invasive burn wound infection:
- infection occurs in unexcised burn and invades viable underlying tissue
- diagnosis may be supported by histologic examination or quantitative cultures

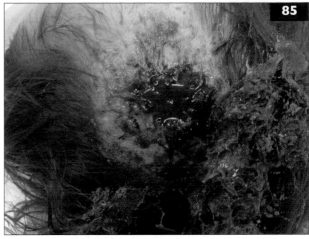

85 Burn impetigo is a superficial loss of epithelium usually seen in healed deep dermal burns and donor sites, caused by *Staphylococcus aureus* and/or *Streptococcus pyogenes*.

gressive intrapulmonary shunting and hypoxia, ileus, nonoliguric renal failure, rising cholestatic chemistries, thrombocytopenia, anuria, vasomotor failure, and death. Treatment involves support of failing organs and a thorough search for occult infection. Wound sepsis is the most virulent infection burn patients suffer, but this is relatively infrequently seen if deep wounds are promptly excised and closed. Prevention of tissue hypoxia by careful hemodynamic support and avoidance of infection by early wound excision and closure are the best strategy to minimize this difficult problem. Prompt and effective surgery is the most effective immunomodulator in acute burn care.

BURN WOUND INFECTION

Until quite recently, overwhelming wound sepsis was a very common cause of death in burn patients. Although early excision and closure of deep wounds have reduced its frequency, it remains a very difficult problem today. A set of burn wound infection definitions includes four subtypes: burn impetigo, open burn-related surgical wound infection, burn wound cellulitis, and invasive burn wound infection (*Table 22*).

Burn impetigo is a superficial loss of epithelium secondary to *Staphylococcus aureus* and/or *Streptococcus pyogenes*, usually seen in recently healed deep dermal burns or donor sites (**85**). Treatment requires wound cleansing, which often mandates shaving of nearby hair-bearing areas with topical and sometimes systemic antistaphylococcal agents. In some cases skin grafting of denuded areas is required.

Open burn-related surgical wound infection describes purulent infection that develops in excised wounds and donor sites. These infections usually drain pus and are associated with systemic toxicity and loss of skin grafts. In many situations these infections are associated with inadequately excised wounds. Treatment requires debridement of necrotic and infected material with delayed wound closure. Staphylococcal toxic shock syndrome has been reported in burn patients and is a risk particularly when occlusive dressings are employed over deep burns.

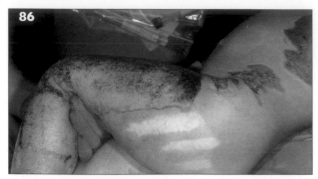

86 Burn wound cellulitis refers to spreading dermal infection in uninjured skin around a burn wound or donor site, usually secondary to *Streptococcus pyogenes*. Note blanched finger impressions.

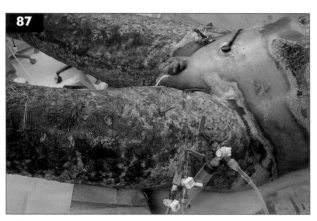

87 Invasive burn wound infection can be an overwhelming threat to life. Patients present with extreme toxicity, high fever, and a hyperdynamic circulatory state followed by bacteremia, hypotension, and cardiovascular collapse. These infections are generally bacterial, most commonly with *Pseudomonas aeruginosa* (as in this patient) or *Staphylococcus aureus*.

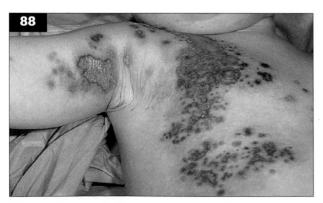

88 Less frequently, fungal or viral infections can develop in burn wounds. This child has a herpetic wound infection. Infection is usually secondary to reactivation.

Burn wound cellulitis (**86**) refers to spreading dermal infection in uninjured skin around a burn wound or donor site, usually secondary to *S. pyogenes*. This can vary from an early subtle erythema a centimeter or so around the wound to a brawny erythema involving an entire limb or torso. It is rare to recover an organism from wound swabs or dermal aspirates. This is most commonly seen in the first few days after a burn, or as a postoperative donor site complication. Prophylactic antibiotics are not useful for reducing this complication.

Invasive burn wound infection (**87**) can be an overwhelming threat to life. Patients present with extreme toxicity, high fever, and a hyperdynamic circulatory state followed by bacteremia, hypotension, and cardiovascular collapse. Three diagnostic techniques are discussed including clinical examination, quantitative cultures of a burn wound biopsy, and burn wound histology. Both quantitative culture and histologic examination are subject to sampling errors and delay in treatment. From a practical perspective, clinical diagnosis of these infections, generally by changes in wound appearance and odor in a toxic patient, suffices. Prompt treatment is essential, and is effected by parenteral and topical antimicrobials, resuscitation from septic shock, and prompt wound excision. These infections are generally bacterial, most commonly with *Pseudomonas aeruginosa* or *S. aureus*. Other organisms, fungi, and viruses (**88**) can be seen, but the degree of systemic toxicity is usually less.

AUSTERE ALTERNATIVES

Most hospitals in the world have very limited access to critical care as it is practiced in the developed world. In some circumstances, this reality must inevitably lead to *de facto* rationing, particularly when patients present with very large burns. Ideally, these decisions are made as a clinical group, perhaps agreeing on a maximum burn size that can be addressed. When possible, transfer agreements to higher levels of care are arranged for those presenting with injuries above this level.

Chapter 8

Definitive Wound Closure

'Lasting change is a series of compromises.'
Jane Goodall (1934– present), British primatologist.

'The greater the ignorance the greater the dogmatism.'
Sir William Osler (1849–1919), Canadian physician.

In this third general phase of burn care, the patient should have bulk physiologic wound closure and be in a more stable systemic state. Surgical objectives are replacement of temporary wound closure membranes with autograft and definitive closure of complex

AN UNMET NEED

While still in training, the Swiss surgeon Jaques Louis Reverdin (1842–1929) is credited with performing the first modern successful skin autograft, for a nonhealing, granulating wound of a thumb, in Geneva in 1869. Reverdin's technique was essentially what would later be called a pinch graft. His inspiration is unknown. A young British surgeon, George David Pollock (1817–1897) of London (who was from a military family and had been raised in India), is credited with the first skin graft to a burn. In 1871, aware of Riverdin's report, he was called to evaluate an 8-year-old girl with a chronic open contracted burn of the thigh. She had suffered the original burn at age 6. He performed four separate operations on Anne T. over the succeeding months, describing the slow closure of her wounds. One attempt was from an unrelated skin donor, which sloughed after several weeks, an early reported attempt at allografting.

Over the next few decades, skin grafts were cut with freehand knives, either as pinch grafts or as sheets cut with long blades. This cannot have been precise. Unhappy with his inability to cut grafts of precise thickness, Earl Padgett, a general surgeon practicing at the University of Kansas, teamed up with George Hood, a University of Kansas mechanical engineer. They realized that to achieve a uniform thickness, they would have to somehow control the location of the skin in relation to the blade. This concept led to the development of the Padgett–Hood hand-powered drum dermatome in the late 1930s, in which the skin is glued to the drum, giving much more control to autograft procurement. The first powered dermatome is credited to the American surgeon Harry M. Brown, who conceived the idea while caring for burned soldiers in a Japanese prison camp during the Second World War.

The concept of precise mechanical meshing allowing graft expansion was conceived and perfected by an American general surgeon, James Carlton Tanner, and a Belgian engineer and plastic surgery resident, Jacques J. Vandeput, in the early 1960s while both worked in Atlanta, Georgia. They developed the first commercial meshing device, the Tanner–Vandeput mesh dermatome. All of these techniques and instruments have evolved, but all began with a vision of an unmet need.

smaller wounds, including the head and neck, hands, feet, and genitalia. From a practical perspective, depending on the patient and their wound, these activities will occur in tandem. However, this is not always the case and it is helpful to separate the activities when planning specific operations. The most pressing need is for definitive bulk wound closure with autograft. Bulk definitive closure is always the first priority, virtually all other needs can wait. What follow are descriptions of practical consensus approaches to these smaller complex wounds.

MASSIVE BURNS

Definitive wound closure in patients with massive burns can be a frustrating and elusive goal. In some patients, cultured materials can provide some element of definitive closure. Hopefully this will become a more practical reality in a few years. For most patients with massive deep injuries, multiple thin reharvests of available donor sites provide the bulk of definitive coverage. However, no donor site can be harvested indefinitely and, in some patients, changing the initial objective from complete to 95% definitive closure allows for a period of rehabilitation and strengthening near the end of the acute stay, prior to embarking on efforts to close the last difficult 5% of their wound. This judgment should me made on a case-by-case basis.

FACIAL BURNS

Your initial work on facial burns will have an important impact on your patients' ability to reintegrate. Burns in this location should be approached in a careful and studied way. Initial objectives are wound closure and facial function. However, these should be achieved with an eye to aesthetics and future reconstructive options. Commonly, compromises must be made between ideal objectives and the availability of acceptable donor material.

Good management decisions are based on an accurate estimation of burn depth. The varying depth and appendage density of the face make these determinations more difficult. The central face is rich in sweat and sebaceous glands, making it likely that even deep second-degree burns will resurface with quite a nice result when they are allowed to heal. The anatomy of the skin in this area makes a conservative initial approach physiologically sound. This is not the case as you move to the forehead and peripheral face. The entire face comprises only 4% of the body surface, so overwhelming sepsis from an unexcised facial burn is vanishingly rare. For these reasons, most active burn surgeons do not perform early excision of facial burns. The more common practice is to let wounds in this area begin to slough in topical care or membrane dressings, clearly demonstrating their depth and likelihood of healing, before approaching full-thickness components at 7 or more days after injury.

Topical care of partial-thickness or indeterminate depth facial burns varies widely among programs. Any strategy that prevents desiccation is reasonable. A large variety of topical medications and membranes are applied to these wounds. None is clearly superior. A common and effective program advises silver sulphadiazine on deeper partial and full-thickness burns and viscous antibiotic-containing ointments on more superficial injuries. Gentle removal of necrotic debris and prevention of desiccation are common to all successful management plans. Burns around the eyes can be dressed with topical ophthalmic antibiotic ointments. Many programs have adopted cautious use of membrane dressings on selected facial burns.

The face can be divided into seven aesthetic units (**89, 90**). It has been taught that facial grafting should be done in aesthetic units. However, this is not appropriate if it requires excision of any more than small amounts of superficial burn or unburned skin. Graft thickness in facial burn grafting usually requires a compromise between the ideal of thick split-thickness or full-thickness grafts with the realities of donor site limitations and donor site morbidity. In general, expanded local flaps are not appropriate acutely. Color match is an important consideration. It has been taught that facial burns are ideally resurfaced with donor skin not previously harvested to maintain normal coloration. However, on many occasions, the match that needs to be made is with healed, depigmented burns (**91**). In this situation, the best color match is provided by reharvested split-thickness donor sites. Excisions are done in a layered fashion. The operations tend to be bloody, but generous subeschar clysis with dilute epinephrine solution and elevation of the head of the operating table significantly reduce blood loss. Sheet grafts are generally applied. These can be left open in cooperative patients, but are better protected with tie-over dressings, particularly in children (**92**). After the grafts have vascularized, massage and pressure therapy should begin immediately.

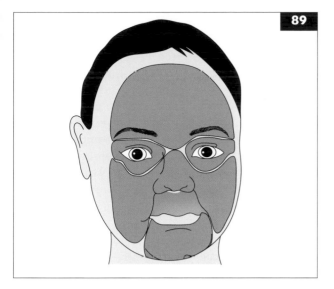

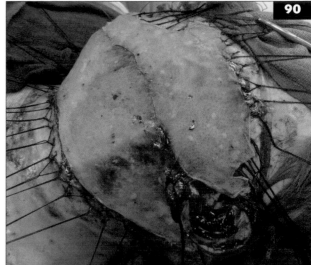

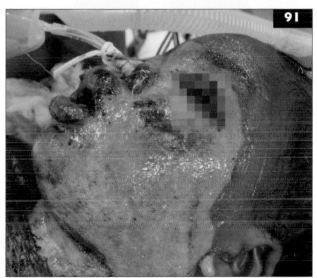

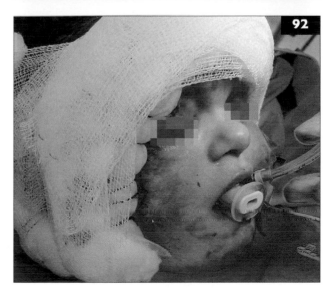

89 For aesthetic purposes, the face can be divided into seven cosmetic units. When possible, these should be resurfaced as units. However, this is an important place for compromise.

90 Many facial burns do not lend themselves to aesthetic unit excision.

91 On many occasions, the match that needs to be made is with healed, depigmented burns. In this situation, the best color match is provided by reharvested split-thickness donor sites.

92 Facial burn excisions are done using a layered technique. These sheet grafts can be left open in cooperative patients, but are better protected with tie-over dressings, particularly in children.

Scar management should start in the early weeks after successful healing of partial-thickness burns or grafted full-thickness injuries. Moisture, massage, and compression are the cornerstones of therapy. Custom fitted clear face masks, some lined with silicone, can be made from a mold or through a helium–neon laser noncontact process (**93**). Increasingly, tuneable dye laser treatments are being added to early postacute scar management if wounds begin to demonstrate significant early hypertrophy (**94**). Areas of tension will predictably exacerbate hypertrophy and can often be alleviated with well-designed Z-plasties (**95**). Ideally, the operating team will follow patients with deep facial burns very closely during the first years after injury to ensure optimal function and appearance. Multimodality treatment of deep facial burns, combining prompt effective surgery, moisture, massage, compression, early functional reconstruction, and Z-plasty, can give excellent long-term aesthetic and functional results (**96, 97**).

EYELID BURNS

The initial objective of early management of burns of and around the eyelids is to evaluate the globe for corneal burn or other injury, to ensure coverage of the globes, and to check for and treat acute intraocular hypertension if present (see **15**). In the first days after injury, lid edema will protect the globe. It is almost never necessary to perform a tarsorrhaphy acutely. Subsequently, eyelid function is most commonly compromised by contracture, which exposes the globe and threatens exposure, keratitis, ulceration, perforation, and blindness. Globe exposure should be watched for. When this is relatively mild, ocular lubricants will suffice. During sleep, Bell's

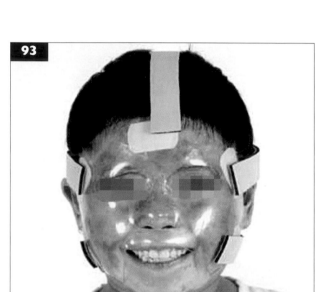

93 Custom fitted clear face masks, some lined with silicone, can be made from a mold or through a helium–neon laser noncontact process.

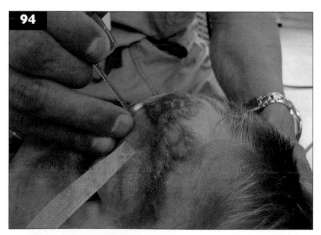

94 Selective use of the tuneable dye laser is a potential adjunct to early postacute scar management if wounds begin to demonstrate significant early hypertrophy. This tool should only be used as part of a program of scar managment.

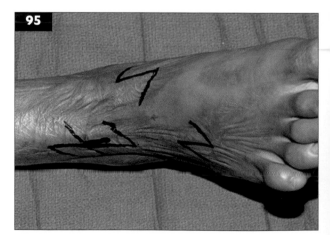

95 Areas of tension will predictably exacerbate hypertrophy and can often be alleviated with well-designed Z-plasties.

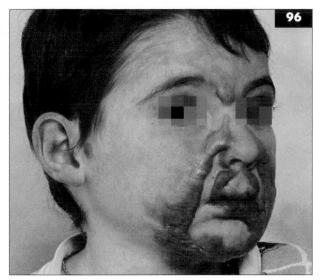

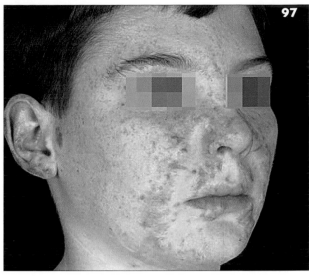

96, 97 Multimodality treatment of deep facial burns, combining prompt effective surgery, moisture, massage, compression, early functional reconstruction, tuneable dye laser therapy, and Z-plasty, can give excellent long-term aesthetic and functional results. These photos are separated by three Z-plasty procedures and six tuneable dye laser treatments over 7 years. (Courtesy of Dr. Mathias B. Donelan.)

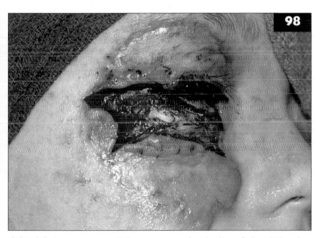

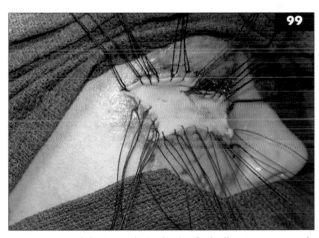

98, 99 In most eyelid ectropia, the bulk of the lid substance is preserved, but needs to be 'unfurled' into a normal position, carefully preserving remant normal anatomy.

phenomenon, a reflex in which the globe rotates in an upward direction such that the subcorneal conjunctiva may be exposed but the corneal epithelium is protected by the contracted upper lid, will help. More severe exposure, particularly if keratitis occurs, should generally be managed with acute lid release and graft (**98, 99**). It is difficult to perform upper and lower lid releases well at the same time. Therefore, the most deformed lid is released first. When doing these

procedures, the remnant normal tarsal plate, orbicularis oculi muscle, levator palpebrae muscle, orbital septum, and palpebral conjunctiva should be carefully protected. In most cases, the normal anatomy simply needs to be 'unfurled'. Thick split-thickness grafts generally suffice for coverage, although full-thickness grafts seem to be more appropriate for lower lids. The lacrimal apparatus should be avoided when releasing lower lids.

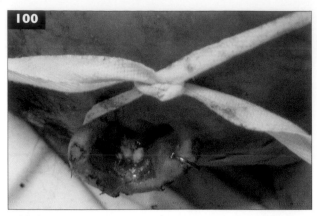

100 It is important to avoid pressure on burned ears to minimize secondary deformity. Ties used to secure endotrachael and nasogastric tubes should be monitored.

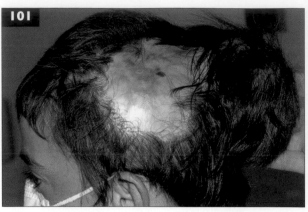

101 Late alopecia can often be much improved with later rotation of expanded hair-bearing flaps.

EAR BURNS

The cartilaginous skeleton of the ear has a poor blood supply and becomes infected easily, with significant adverse aesthetic results. Initial management of ear burns attempts to lower the incidence of auricular chondritis by application of mafenide acetate to all but superficial burns, as this will penetrate the underlying cartilage and reduce the incidence of infection. It is also important to avoid pressure on burned ears to minimize secondary deformity (**100**). Subsequent management is based on depth of injury: if the injury is deep, debridement of necrotic skin and cartilage is followed by thin split-thickness autograft closure. Grafts can be secured with fine absorbable suture or with cyanoacrylic glue. A variety of devices can be fashioned for postoperative protection.

SCALP BURNS

In children and adults, hair follicles of the scalp tend to be thick and deep, protecting epithelial cells that can resurface most mid and deep dermal burns. This argues for an initial nonexcisional approach to most scalp burns unless they are remarkably deep. Shaving burned scalp will facilitate cleansing, topical care, and wound evaluation. Thick dermis and density of appendages make unburned scalp a durable donor site, except in very young children, whose hair follicles are more superficial. When harvesting the scalp, an awareness of the location of the anterior hair line in small children with their high bossed foreheads, will prevent inadvertent harvesting of the forehead with adverse cosmetic consequences. Leaving a fringe of unshaved hair at the anterior hairline will help prevent this complication. Areas requiring grafting will demonstrate late alopecia, which can often be much improved with later rotation of expanded hair-bearing flaps (**101**).

NECK BURNS

Unequivocal full-thickness neck burns are ideally excised and grafted with thick sheet autograft early in the patient's course. Grafts are well secured with large tie-over dressings (**102**). Postoperative care focuses on maintaining the breadth of the graft, which has a tendency to contract when the neck is held in a neutral or flexed position. Conforming neck splints, graft massage, and an extended supine sleeping position will help. Patients requiring tracheostomy can have this done through fresh grafts. In some cases, early contraction of neck burns or grafts will compromise airway access and patient comfort, and early neck release is then indicated.

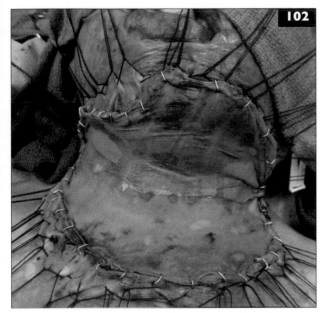

102 Postoperative neck grafts are secured with tie-over dressings. Postoperative intubation is almost never required.

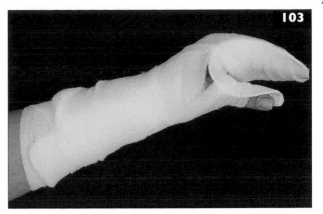

103 Hand splinted in a position of function, with the metacarpophalangeal joints at 70–90°, the interphalangeal joints in extension, the first web space open, and the wrist at 20° of extension.

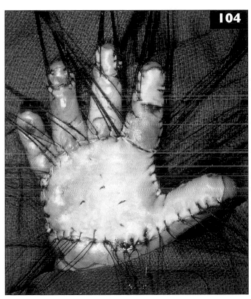

104 Deep dermal and full thickness burns should undergo prompt excision and sheet autograft closure. With aggressive postoperative hand therapy, functional outcomes are excellent.

HAND BURNS

Like facial burns, hand burns have an impact on outcome far out of proportion to their size. They should be a particular focus from the outset of care, so as not to compromise long-term hand function. The most important early objective is to ensure that hand perfusion is not compromised by near circumferential eschar or elevated compartment pressures. Burned hands should be regularly examined for tissue turgor, temperature, and the presence of pulsatile Doppler flow in the digital pulp. If there is any question of compromised flow, prompt escharotomy and/or fasciotomy should be done (see **19**).

Hands should be elevated to minimize edema and ranged twice daily. Ranging through a full range of motion twice daily is optimal. At other times hands can be splinted in a position of function, with the metacarpophalangeal joints at 70–90°, the interphalangeal joints in extension, the first web space open, and the wrist at 20° of extension (**103**). Deep dermal and full thickness burns should undergo prompt excision and sheet autograft closure (**104**). Because of the thick skin of the palm, most palmar burns will heal, but deep dermal or full-thickness injuries are best grafted, generally with thick split-thickness grafts. At 7 days after surgery, passive and, if possible, active hand therapy should begin. Even very destructive hand burns should be managed with an expectation of a functional result consistent with activities of daily living. Essential components of this functional goal are to maintain flexion at the metacarpophalangeal (MCP) joints and opposition between the remnant of the thumb and digits.

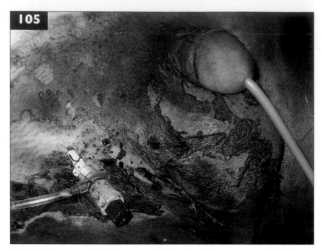

105 Most genital burns will heal without surgery, but when needed, full-thickness burns of the scrotum and phallus can be successfully grafted with quite excellent outcomes.

GENITAL BURNS

Although early excision has been advocated, full-thickness injuries to the genitalia are generally best left to slough spontaneously while other issues are addressed. This physiologically small and well-perfused area is rarely the source of threatening sepsis, and redundant genital skin is remarkably capable of contracting and compensating for significant loss of surface area. Full-thickness burns of the scrotum and phallus can be successfully grafted when needed with quite excellent outcomes (**105**). Meatal stenosis will occasionally occur after a burn to the glans, and is easily rectified with meatotomy. Finally, fecal diversion is virtually never necessary to manage deep burns of the genitalia, perineum, or perianal area successfully.

AUSTERE ALTERNATIVES

In most austere environments, allograft and other temporary membranes are not available, due either to expense or to supply issues. Surgeons may be faced with situations in which patients are too unstable, burns are too large, or equipment needed to procure skin grafts is not available to allow for immediate autografting of burns. In this setting, the choice is to allow all or part of a wound to liquefy and separate, or to leave some or all of an excised wound open. It may be necessary to delay definite closure by autografting. If burns are clearly deep, it seems preferable to remove necrotic tissue and leave wounds open, rather than to let the eschar liquefy and separate. These clean granulating wounds can be autografted at a later date (**106**). If some autograft is available, it is best to graft those areas that will reliably take graft, ensuring some closure, while leaving open difficult areas, such as proximal joints of the extremities or the back.

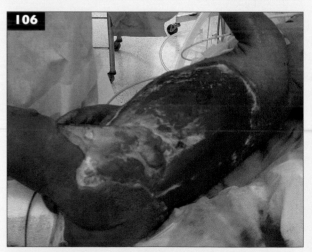

106 If immediate autografting is not possible, and temporary membranes are not available, excised wounds will generally granulate, allowing later autografting. Although not ideal, this is preferable to allowing unexcised eschar to liquefy and separate.

CHAPTER 9

SPECIAL INJURIES AND ILLNESSES

'Common sense in medicine is the master workman.'
Peter Mere Latham (1789–1875),
Londoner, physician extraordinary to
Queen Victoria 1837–1875.

'The most difficult thing of all to see is that which is right in front of your eyes.'
Johann Wolfgang von Goethe (1749–1832),
German writer and philosopher.

Burn units provide excellent care for a number of special clinical problems that benefit from the combination of wound and critical care expertise available in these programs. These situations include high-voltage electrical injuries, chemical burns, burns from tar and other thermoplastic road materials, cold injuries, TEN, purpura fulminans, soft tissue injuries, soft tissue infections, and injuries caused by abuse or neglect. Each of these conditions has specific unique initial priorities to consider (*Table 23*).

Table 23 Unique initial priorities of nonburn problems appropriate for burn unit care

Electrical injuries
- Cardiac rhythm should be monitored in high- (>1000 volt) and selected intermediate- (220–1000 volt) voltage exposures for 12–24 hr
- Low- and intermediate-voltage exposures can cause locally destructive injuries, but uncommonly result in systemic sequelae
- Delayed neurologic and ocular sequelae can occur after high-voltage injury, so neurologic and ocular examinations should be documented during initial assessment
- Extremities in the path of high-voltage current should be monitored for compartment syndrome and be decompressed promptly when it develops
- Bladder catheters should be placed in all patients suffering high-voltage exposure to document and help manage pigmenturia

Chemical burns
- Irrigate cutaneous wounds with tap water for at least 30 minutes for acidic exposures
- If alkaline exposure, irrigate until wound does not have a soapy feel or pH is normalized
- Irrigate the globe with isotonic crystalloid. Blepharospasm may require ocular anesthetic administration
- Concentrated hydrofluoric acid exposures may be complicated by life-threatening hypocalcemia. Serum calcium must be closely monitored and supplemented. Subeschar infiltration of 10% calcium gluconate solution may be appropriate after exposure to highly concentrated or anhydrous solutions
- Dilute hydrofluoric acid exposures are treated with topical 2.5% calcium gluconate gel until pain is resolved. Hands may be placed into a glove filled with gel

Tar burns
- Tars should be cooled with tap water irrigation initially
- Wounds can be dressed in lipophilic solvent topical agents to facilitate removal

(Continued overleaf)

Table 23 Unique initial priorities of nonburn problems appropriate for burn unit care (continued)

Toxic epidermal necrolysis

- TEN is a diffuse cutaneous and visceral epidermal slough at the dermal–epidermal junction, usually associated with an antecedent flu-like syndrome and often with drug administration
- The severity of cutaneous, mucous membrane, and conjunctival involvement varies widely. Typically, visceral slough follows days behind cutaneous involvement
- Differentiation from drug eruptions, viral exanthems, or SSS can occasionally be difficult on examination. Skin biopsy may be helpful in equivocal cases
- Treatment involves prevention of wound desiccation and infection, treatment of septic complications, and support of failing organ systems, while awaiting re-epithelialization
- Early ophthalmologic care is important to optimal long-term outcome
- Those with severe oropharyngeal or tracheobronchial involvement may require intubation for airway protection and enteral tube feedings for nutritional support

Purpura fulminans

- Typically a complication of meningococcal sepsis
- Probably secondary to transient protein C deficiency. Fresh frozen plasma or activated protein C should be considered early
- Frequently accompanied by organ failure
- Treatment involves management of organ failure and excision and grafting of wounds to prevent wound sepsis
- Can be associated with adrenal infarction or hemorrhage and acute adrenal insufficiency
- Long-term morbidity secondary to major amputation and epiphyseal arrest is common

Staphylococcal scalded skin syndrome

- SSS is a reaction to a staphylococcal exotoxin which results in epithelial separation at the granular layer
- May be related only to colonization, rather than frank infection
- Most common in infants and young children
- Superficial wounds heal quickly if infection and desiccation do not occur
- Mucous membrane and conjunctival involvement is not seen. This is a key point of physical exam and diagnostic differentiation
- Empiric anti-staphylococcal antibiotics should be administered while a focus of infection is eliminated

Soft tissue infection

- Essential first steps are suspicion, exploration of suspicious compartments, and aggressive excision of nonviable or infected tissue
- Antibiotics are important, but are adjuncts to surgery
- Hyperbaric oxygen can be considered as an adjunct to anerobic soft tissue infections, but surgery is cornerstone of management

Soft tissue trauma

- Large soft tissue wounds or degloving injuries are well-managed in the burn unit
- Careful trauma-specific secondary survey is important
- Tertiary survey evaluation for missed injuries is important

Injuries of abuse

- Should be considered in all injured patients, not only children. Burns are common in domestic violence
- Suspicious injuries must be filed with the appropriate state agency
- Important points of examination include uniformity of burn depth, absence of splash marks, sharply defined wound margins, porcelain contact sparing, flexor sparing, stocking or glove patterns, dorsal location of contact burns of the hand, and localized very deep contact burns
- Important points of history include unusual or conflicting stories, prior injuries, and delayed presentation
- Patients should be admitted for evaluation, even if the injury itself is of little physiologic significance
- Screening long bone series and CT scanning of the head for occult injuries should be considered

ELECTRICAL INJURIES

Electrical injuries can be divided into high (>1000 volt), intermediate (120–1000 volt), and low (<120 volt) exposures (Textbox: Which is more dangerous, AC or DC?). It is uncommon to see compartment syndromes, arrhythmias, loss of consciousness, or myoglobinuria in patients exposed to low and intermediate range voltages. However, these complications are quite common in those sustaining high-voltage injuries, and should be specifically sought. High-voltage electrocutions are also very commonly accompanied by blunt trauma because of associated falls.

Patients sustaining good electrical contact with mid-range, and even low-voltage sources can sustain quite destructive local injuries, but rarely have these other associated complications. This type of deep localized hand injury is common in electricians (**107**). Small deep injuries are often well-managed

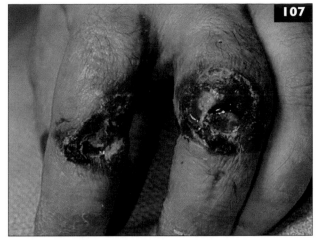

107 Deep localized hand injuries are common in electricians. Small deep injuries are often well-managed with topical care awaiting spontaneous slough and healing by contraction and epithelialization. Local or distant flaps are sometimes an attractive option in patients with larger deep injuries.

WHICH IS MORE DANGEROUS, AC OR DC?

In 1881, Albert Southwick, a Buffalo New York dentist, saw an intoxicated elderly man touch the terminals of an electrical generator, and noted how quickly and painlessly the man died. He described this episode to his state senator who proposed that electrocution replace hanging for New York state executions. Meanwhile, Thomas Edison was setting up a direct current (DC) utility to light New York's cities. George Westinghouse's alternating current (AC) technology threatened Edison's monopoly. Stepped-up AC is cheaper to transmit over distances, so Edison focused his anti-AC campaign on the relative safety of DC. He published a series of experiments showing multiple species of animals are killed with far lower AC voltages than DC, until he was stopped by the Society for the Prevention of Cruelty to Animals. Meanwhile, in 1888, the New York Legislature passed Chapter 489 of the Laws of New York, establishing New York as the first state to execute by electrocution. Edison hoped to use the fact of AC electrocution to help him publicize the relative safety of DC. Employees of Edison's lab at Menlo Park were involved in purchasing Westinghouse AC generators for the prison system and facilitating designs. Meanwhile, in 1889, William Kemmler killed his lover with an axe in Buffalo, and was sentenced to death by electrocution. George Westinghouse, hoping to protect AC's reputation, funded Kemmler's appeal, while Edison was a witness for the State. The appeal was denied and, on August 6 1890, Kemmler was executed by AC electric chair, on the second attempt. George Westinghouse witnessed the execution and publicly stated, '*They would have done better with an axe.*' Edison's supporting experimental work clearly demonstrated that DC is safer, but the economics of long-distance AC transmission won out in the utility industry. Even Thomas Edison became a convert, and General Electric, the company that evolved from his early work, became, and remains, a world leader in AC technology.

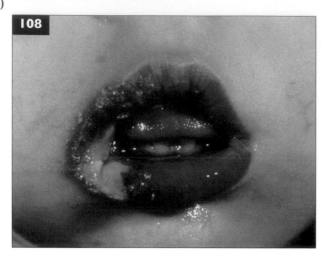

108 Commisure burns in children are best managed conservatively, awaiting eschar separation and spontaneous healing, delaying any reconstruction as they will often heal surprisingly well. Parents are advised to be alert for bleeding, which can occur with separation of the eschar.

with topical care awaiting spontaneous slough and healing by contraction and epithelialization. Another important exception to the early excisional debridement approach is in the child with a commissure burn (**108**), commonly seen in children who have mouthed the junction of an appliance and an extension cord. These wounds are best managed conservatively, awaiting eschar separation and spontaneous healing, delaying any reconstruction as they will often heal surprisingly well. Parents are advised to be alert for bleeding, which can occur with separation of the eschar. If it occurs, bleeding is controlled with pressure between the forefinger and thumb, while en route to the hospital. In patients with larger deep wounds, early excisional debridement and skin graft or flap coverage is a more attractive option. Negative-pressure dressings as an adjunct after excisional debridement can greatly facilitate granulation and subsequent autografting of deep wounds in this setting (**109**).

High-voltage injuries are much more commonly associated with nonwound complications including loss of consciousness, cardiac arrhythmias, falls, fractures, myoglobinuria, compartment syndromes, and delayed neurologic and ocular sequelae. These patients should initially be approached as trauma patients, as there may otherwise be a disturbing number of missed injuries. After appropriate airway and vascular access have been achieved, a systematic trauma secondary survey should be done, with a directed effort to look for visceral injuries, long bone and spine fractures, myoglobinuria, and compartment syndromes. Patients should undergo cardiac monitoring and enzyme screens should be

considered. Depending on the mechanism of injury, CT scanning should be liberally performed (**110**).

Fluid resuscitation requirements are difficult to predict in high-voltage injuries, as the external surface burn does not reflect overall tissue injury. These patients often have a mix of flame burns from clothing ignition, flash burns from electrical arc, deep entry wounds, multiple exit wounds, and deep localized wounds at sites of arc across flexed extremities (**111**). Resuscitation is generally begun based on the size of the surface burn and is very carefully monitored, with additional fluid given as dictated by the standard resuscitation endpoints. Clinically important myoglobinuria is indicated by visibly pigmented urine and is managed in most patients by administration of added crystalloid to an endpoint of a urine output of 2 ml/kg/hr until the urine clears (**112**). In patients with particularly heavily pigmented urine, the addition of sodium bicarbonate to intravenous fluids may facilitate pigment clearance. The occasional patient who does not respond to additional crystalloid with a prompt increase in urine output may respond to mannitol. However, this maneuver reduces the value of urine output as a valid indicator of circulating volume and should therefore be used cautiously. Central venous pressure should ideally be monitored in this situation.

Evolving compartment syndromes are best detected by serial physical examination. Compartment pressure measurements can be helpful in equivocal cases, with pressures over 30 cmH$_2$O considered high. Not all extremities exposed to high voltage require decompression, but at-risk extremities not decompressed require careful monitoring over the first 48 hr.

109 Negative-pressure dressings after excisional debridement can greatly facilitate granulation and subsequent autografting of deep wounds after electrical injury.

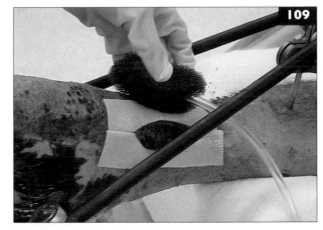

110 Depending on mechanism of injury, CT scanning should be liberally performed in those suffering high-voltage trauma. This epidural hematoma was nearly missed in a school-aged child with a high-voltage injury. An astute physician detected subtle signs of neurologic dysfunction during the initial evaluation, prompting early CT scanning and detection of the enlarging hematoma, which might not otherwise have been detected in the intubated, sedated child until too late to prevent tragic sequelae.

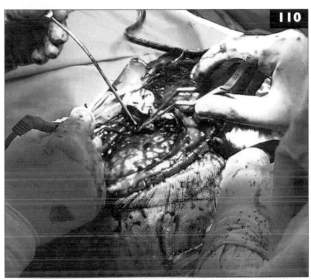

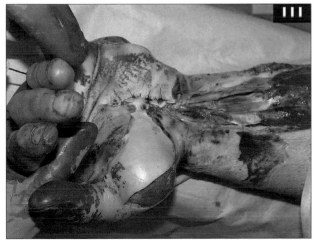

112 Clinically important myoglobinuria is indicated by visibly pigmented urine and is managed in most patients by administration of added crystalloid to an endpoint of a urine output of 2 ml/kg/hr until the urine clears.

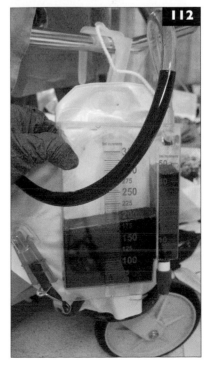

111 Patients suffering high-voltage wounds often have a mix of flame burns from clothing ignition, flash burns from electrical arc, deep entry wounds, multiple exit wounds, and deep localized wounds at sites of current arc across flexed extremities. This patient's wounds illustrate the consequences of arc between points of flexion.

If fasciotomy of tense extremities is not done, the resulting ischemia can cause more tissue injury than the original electrical current.

Definitive closure of these wounds varies with the individual patient, the basic principle being prompt debridement of necrotic material and closure of wounds (**113**). Negative-pressure dressings are useful adjuncts to staged debridment. Any associated cutaneous burns are grafted. Particularly destructive burns may require staged autografting, complex flap closure, or amputation. Keeping an eye on ultimate function is essential. Some patients will develop delayed neurologic deficits and occasionally cataracts, so setting up a long-term follow-up plan is important.

CHEMICAL BURNS

Initial care for most chemical burns is immediate removal of clothing, including jewelry and shoes, and dusting off any powders. Emergency personnel should protect themselves with gloves and aprons. Irrigation with tap water should be done for at least 30 minutes. Alkaline substances are less soluble in water and often take longer to irrigate. The completeness of irrigation can be tested by rubbing gloved fingers together after contact is made with the wound. Residual alkali imparts a soapy feel. Litmus paper can also be used to verify the completeness of irrigation. Some chemicals will be absorbed and have systemic consequences. When in doubt, consultation with a poison control center should be considered. There is no role for neutralization of acid or alkali burn because these reactions generate heat which can further deepen the injury. In patients with ocular exposures, reflexive blepharospasm make it impossible to irrigate the eye adequately. This can be facilitated by topical ocular anesthetics. Patients with large injuries may require fluid resuscitation, initially based on visible surface burn size. Some volatile chemicals are associated with a noxious fume which can compromise the airway.

Hydrofluoric acid is only weakly acidic, but the fluoride anion is very permeable to skin and binds proteins and divalent cations (most importantly calcium). It coagulates proteins and causes a deep corrosive injury. Concentrated hydrofluoric acid exposures can cause very destructive local injuries and are associated with life-threatening acute hypocalcemia. They can be initially managed with subeschar 10% calcium gluconate, monitoring and supplementation of serum calcium and, in some situations, emergent wound excision. There is a very limited role for proximal intra-arterial infusion or Bier-block with calcium gluconate. Hydrofluoric acid is more commonly used for industrial cleaning, rust removal, and etching silicon in a dilute form. Dilute hydrofluoric acid exposures typically present with delayed pain, most often in the fingers, and can generally be managed with irrigation, monitoring, and topical 2.5% calcium gluconate gel.

HOT TAR BURNS

Road construction materials are formulated to remain solid in the hot sun. They must be heated to 300–700°F (~150–370°C) before they will liquify for application. These hot viscous liquids stick to exposed skin and typically cause deep burns (**114**). Immediate management involves cooling with copious tap water irrigation. Subsequently, wounds can be soaked in a lipophilic solvent, such as most viscous antibiotic ointments, to soften the tar prior to removal. The underlying burns are generally quite deep and often require grafting.

COLD INJURIES

Cold injuries are described by a confusing clutter of terms. All still cold or frozen parts should initially undergo moist rewarming in water at approximately 104°F (40°C) (**115**). Injured parts should then be elevated and protected from further injury. After a period of topical wound care to allow for clear demarcation of the necrotic tissue, nonviable tissue is excised and the injured part reconstructed with a combination of primary closure, split-thickness autograft, and local or distant flaps. There is sometimes a progressive microvascular thrombosis caused by endothelial disruption that makes initial determination of injury depth difficult. Patients should be evaluated for systemic hypothermia. In rare patients with brief ischemia time who have profoundly ischemic extremities after thaw, thrombolytic therapy may contribute to limb salvage.

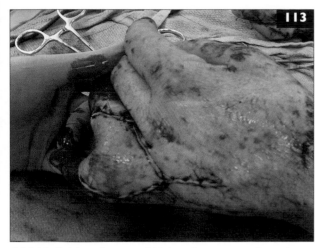

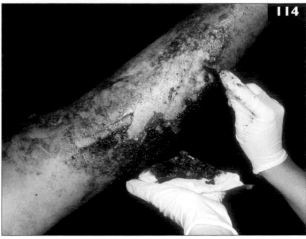

113 Definitive closure of high-voltage wounds varies with the individual patient, the basic principle being prompt debridement of necrotic material and closure of wounds. Any associated cutaneous burns are grafted. Particularly destructive burns may require staged autografting, complex flap closure, or amputation. Keeping an eye on ultimate function is essential. This photo illustrates a radial forearm flap closing a complex high-voltage hand wound.

114 Hot road tar is viscous and will stick to exposed skin typically causing a deep burn. After cooling, wounds can be soaked in a lipophilic solvent, such as most viscous antibiotic ointments, to soften the tar prior to removal. The underlying burns are generally deep.

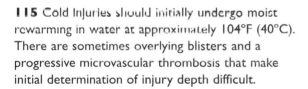

115 Cold injuries should initially undergo moist rewarming in water at approximately 104°F (40°C). There are sometimes overlying blisters and a progressive microvascular thrombosis that make initial determination of injury depth difficult.

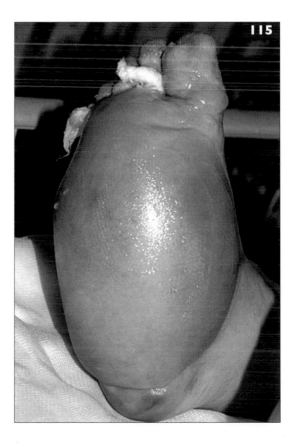

TOXIC EPIDERMAL NECROLYSIS

Toxic epidermal necrolysis (TEN) is also described by a confusing group of names, most commonly erythema multiforme major, Lyell's syndrome, or Steven–Johnson syndrome. It is a systemic inflammatory process triggered in susceptible individuals by a medication or viral syndrome which results in diffuse epidermal separation at the dermal–epidermal junction. Each case seems different in the degree of cutaneous, mucosal, and visceral slough. These areas do not seem to slough synchronously. Typically, a cutaneous rash coalesces into a cutaneous wound initially (**116, 117**). This is followed by the development of conjunctival, mucous membrane, and visceral wounds to a highly variable extent. Most patients with severe slough are managed in burn units, as the combination of wound and critical care expertise has been shown to benefit them. The differential diagnosis includes viral exanthems, staphylococcal scalded skin syndrome, and drug eruptions. Diagnosis is generally clinical, with conjunctival and oral involvement being important features of TEN. In equivocal cases, skin biopsy may be helpful, but sampling error must be considered in such a heterogeneous condition. Although the cutaneous slough causes significant pain and septic complications, the more troublesome wounds are mucosal and visceral (**118**). The pain of the oral ulcerations can be so intense that airway protection with endotrachael intubation is required (**119**).

Principle components of therapy include airway protection as needed, wound care which prevents desiccation and infection, nutritional support, close monitoring for septic complications, and vigilant eye care. Specifics vary with particular programs. Airway protection is required if oral ulcerations make aspiration a risk or if tracheal slough leads to respiratory failure and pneumonia. Wound care can include topical medications such as aqueous silver nitrate or carefully monitored membrane dressings such as porcine xenograft or silver impregnated membranes. Nutritional support is essential and is ideally provided enterally. Some patients will develop pancreatitis from obstruction of sloughed pancreatic ducts or ileus from sloughed intestine and may require periods of parenteral support. Septic complications are very common from cutaneous or visceral sources. Eye care includes lubrication with topical ophthalmic antibiotics and gentle disruption of inflammatory adhesions between the denuded palpebral conjunctiva and cornea. Long-term follow-up is essential, as a significant minority of patients will develop keratitis sicca, corneal neovascularization (**120**), residual skin and nail deformities (**121**), or rarely mucosal strictures.

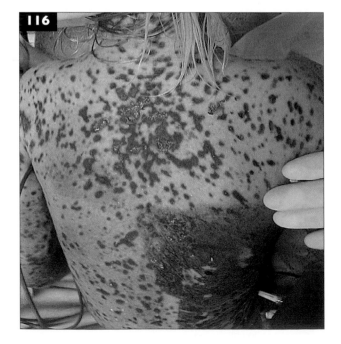

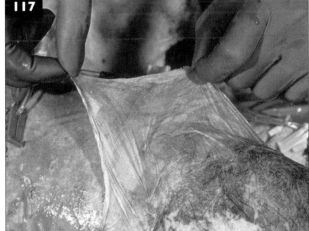

116, 117 TEN patients typically present initially with a flu-like syndrome and cutaneous rash which coalesces into a cutaneous wound. This is followed by the development of conjunctival, mucous membrane, and visceral wounds to a highly variable extent.

118 Although the cutaneous slough causes significant pain and septic complications, the more troublesome wounds in TEN are mucosal and visceral.

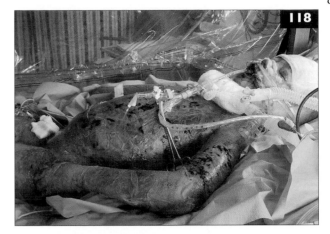

119 The pain of the oral ulcerations in TEN can be so intense that airway protection with endotrachael intubation is required.

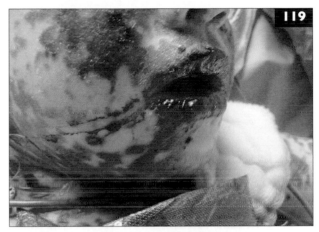

120 Patients with TEN can develop troublesome long-term eye sequelae including keratitis sicca and corneal neovascularization.

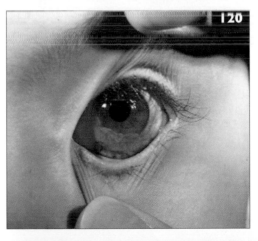

121 Patients with TEN can develop troublesome long-term nail and mucous membrane deformities, as seen here.

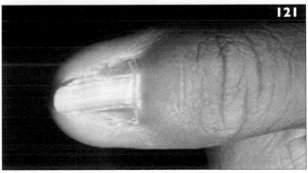

PURPURA FULMINANS

Purpura fulminans is a rare complication of meningococcal or occasionally other bacteremia in which large areas of skin and soft tissue undergo necrosis secondary to microvascular thrombosis, which may be secondary to transient sepsis-induced protein C deficiency (**122–124**). These patients are usually children or young adults and commonly have sepsis-associated organ failure. This combination of problems generally benefits from burn unit care. After initial stabilization, wound excision will facilitate control of sepsis. The proper use of anticoagulants, activated protein C, vasodilators, and thrombolytic agents in these desperately ill patients remains unclear. There is an unfortunate high incidence of extremity loss that favors long-term involvement by the burn program to achieve optimal functional and aesthetic results. Thankfully the syndrome is less common with meningococcal vaccination.

STAPHYLOCOCCAL SCALDED SKIN SYNDROME

Staphylococcal scalded skin syndrome (SSS) is an unusual reaction to a staphylococcal exotoxin which causes a diffuse cutaneous epithelial separation at the granular layer (**125**). It is often associated only with staphylococcal colonization with a phage type producing the exotoxin, rather than actual infection. It is seen most commonly in infants and young children. The wounds are very superficial and tend to heal quickly if infection and desiccation do not occur. An important point of differential diagnosis is the absence of mucous membrane or conjunctival involvement. Empiric antistaphylococcal antibiotics should be administered while a focus of colonization or infection is sought.

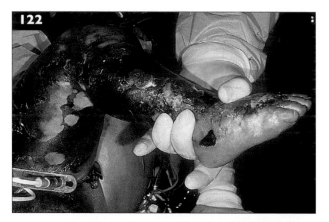

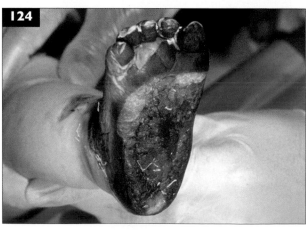

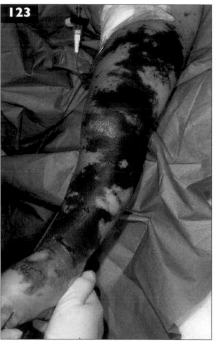

122–124 Purpura fulminans is a rare complication of meningococcal or pneumococcal bacteremia. After initial stabilization, wound excision will facilitate control of sepsis. Vaccination programs have reduced its incidence.

SOFT TISSUE TRAUMA AND INFECTION

Patients with extensive soft tissue injuries or infections are increasingly managed in burn programs. After initial stabilization, wound exploration and aggressive removal of nonviable tissue are the keys to successful management of both problems. These patients often have associated trauma or sepsis-induced organ failure. For soft tissue trauma patients, a careful search for associated injuries is critical (**126**). For soft tissue infection patients, excisional debridement is the primary therapy (**127**). Antibiotics are important adjuncts. Hyperbaric oxygen is a controversial treatment, and can only be recommended as adjunctive therapy in anerobic infection.

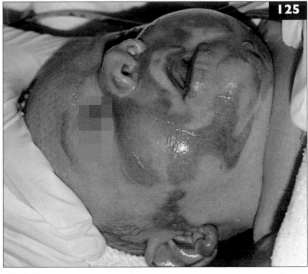

125 Staphylococcal scalded skin syndrome is usually seen in infants and young children. It is a superficial diffuse cutaneous slough with no mucosal or conjunctival involvement, secondary to a staphyoloccal exotoxin. With good wound care, healing tends to be rapid and recovery complete.

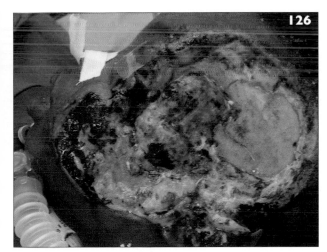

126 For soft tissue trauma patients, a careful search for associated injuries is critical. This child was dragged by a car, suffering complex wounds and associated trauma.

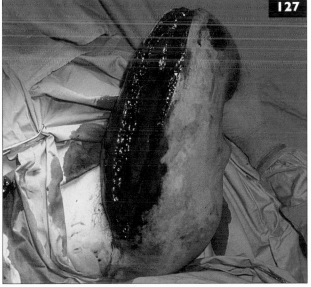

127 For soft tissue infection patients, excisional debridement is the primary treatment. This patient, with Group-A streptococcal myositis, presented with overwhelming systemic sepsis and relatively subtle local signs of muscle involvement. Exploration revealed extensive necrosis and infection of his triceps which was excised promptly. He went on to survive his infection.

INJURIES OF ABUSE

The possibility of abuse or neglect should be part of the evaluation considered when evaluating every burn patient. As many as 20% of pediatric burns have been reported to be the result of abuse or neglect, but such injuries also occur in adults, particularly in settings of domestic violence. Suspicious injuries must be filed with the appropriate state agency. Important information to gather and consider include tap water temperature, duration of contact, caretakers involved, documentation of conflicting reports from involved caretakers, delay in seeking treatment, and prior injuries. Important points of examination to consider include uniformity of burn depth, absence of splash marks, sharply defined wound margins, porcelain contact sparing, flexor sparing (**128**), stocking or glove patterns (**129**), dorsal location of contact burns of the hand and localized very deep contact burns (**130**). Such patients should be admitted to the hospital for evaluation even if the injury itself is of little physiologic significance. Screening long bone series and CT scanning of the head for occult injuries should be considered in at-risk children.

COMBINED BURNS AND TRAUMA

Some patients will present with combined burns and nonburn trauma. Sometimes, the burn priorities conflict with the trauma priorities. Each patient is different and they tend to present unique management decisions that require thoughtful compromise (**131, 132**). Common problems and solutions are outlined in *Table 24*.

Table 24 Common management conflicts in combined burn and trauma patients

Situation	Conflicts	Resolutions
Coincident burn and head injury	Burn resuscitation may exacerbate cerebral edema. Intracranial pressure monitors may become infected if placed through a burn	Tightly control fluid resuscitation. Minimize use of intracranial pressure monitors
Coincident burn and lung injury	Chest tubes placed through burns can result in empyema	Try to place tubes through unburned skin. Minimize use and duration of chest tubes
Coincident burn and rib fractures	Epidural catheters provide good analgesia for rib fractures, but may become infected if placed through a burn	Rely on parenteral pain medication. Use epidurals for shortest possible duration and try to place catheters through unburned skin
Coincident burn and unknown abdominal injury	Overlying burn and hyperdynamic physiology can obscure intraabdominal injuries	Liberal use of CT and FAST based on mechanism of injury
Coincident burn and documented abdominal solid-organ injury	Monitoring of nonoperative management of solid organ injuries is difficult with simultaneous burn resuscitation, particularly if there is overlying burn	Careful monitoring, serial FAST, operate on more severe injuries
Coincident fractured and burned extremities	Internal fixation through burn risks deep infection; casting burned limbs risks wound sepsis	Early external fixation and autografting of injured extremities. Internal fixation is reasonable if it is done through unburned skin

128 Flexor sparing is a suspicious pattern often associated with forceful immersion injury.

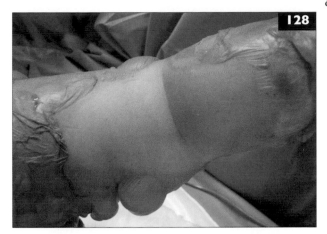

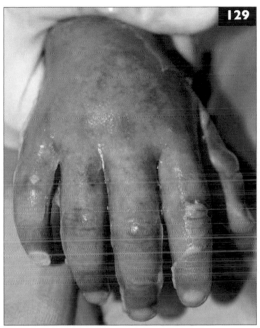

129 Stocking or glove patterns can also be suspicious for forced immersion.

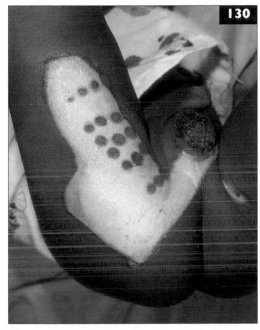

130 Unusual shape or location of contact burns should prompt suspicion of nonaccidental injury.

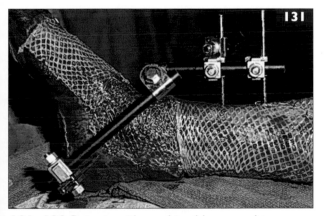

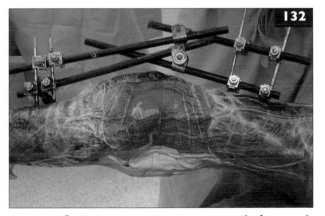

131, 132 Patients with combined burns and trauma can present conflicting priorities in management. In fractured and burned extremities, a combination of external fixation, early grafting, and vacuum-assisted closure is reasonable. In other settings, early amputation is advisable.

AUSTERE ALTERNATIVES

In austere and military environments, combined burns and trauma are common. There are a predictable set of conflicting priorities (*Table 9.2*). In the developing world, occupational safety measures and emergency services are not as evolved as in the developed world (**133**). Management will be limited by available imaging, critical care, and operative resources. Burned fractured extremities are ideally externally fixed, excised, and autografted. In some situations, immediate amputation may be the more practical course. Injuries of abuse occur all over the world. In developing countries, social services are less evolved, putting practitioners in the difficult situation of judging how best to manage the social situation and to whom to discharge patients.

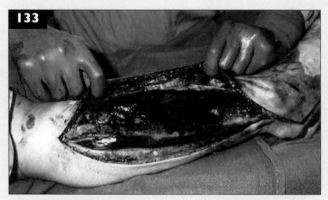

133 High-voltage and other injuries are more common in the developing world, as safety measures are often less robust. Long-term disability related to these injuries is of greater consequence in localities where social services are less evolved. This patient suffered a high-voltage injury. Prompt decompression of the leg may contribute to limb salvage.

CHAPTER 10

OUT-PATIENT MANAGEMENT

'Home's the most excellent place of all.'
Neil Diamond (1941– present),
singer, in 'Heartlight'.

'Soap and water and common sense are the best disinfectants.'
Sir William Osler (1849–1919), Canadian physician.

Most small burns are very well managed in the out-patient setting. Even patients with larger wounds can have substantial portions of their later care delivered in the out-patient setting. In theory, with the proper family training and support, very significant patient needs can be met at home (Textbox: Limits of care at home). Ideally, there is a seamless interface between the in-patient and out-patient components of a burn program. Out-patient burn management can be difficult, and if done poorly can result in needless suffering. Clear and consistent planning is very helpful (*Table 25* [overleaf]).

LIMITS OF CARE AT HOME

In 1809, in Motley's Glen Kentucky, Jane Todd Crawford, a prosperous pioneer farmer's wife thought she was pregnant. Her steady and massive enlargement confused local doctors so they sent for Ephraim McDowell of Danville, some 60 miles away. He arrived on horseback on December 13th, made the diagnosis of a large abdominal tumor, and suggested operation. Elective abdominal surgery was not practiced at that time. Born in Virginia from a Scots–Irish family in 1771, Ephraim McDowell moved with his father to wilderness Kentucky at the age of 13. He attended school nearby and was later apprenticed to a physician back in Virginia. He then attended Edinburgh University, learning much about the limited surgery of the time, primarily stone extraction, obstetrics, and trauma care. He returned to Danville, Kentucky in 1795 and quickly became popular and busy, marrying the daughter of Kentucky's first governor. Desiring to recover, Mrs. Crawford took Dr. McDowell's suggestion and rode to his home, supporting her abdomen on the saddle. In a 25 min operation in his kitchen, he performed the first successful removal of an ovarian tumor (22 pounds), while she recited Psalms. She convalesced in his house. On the 5th day she was up and on the 25th day she remounted her horse and rode back to her home and family, living another 32 years. Dr. McDowell slowed down in his later years to enjoy time on his farm near Lexington, and died in 1830. Dr. McDowell modeled the comprehensive surgical care idealized today.

Table 25 Considerations in out-patient burn care

Patient
- The airway must not be at risk
- Fluid resuscitation is not required
- The patient can eat and drink
- Community and family support is adequate for monitoring, wound care, and transportation
- The patient and family must understand the care plan
- There is no suspicion of abuse
- The wound unequivocally does not require surgery

Techniques
- Teach the patient and the family
- Set up a clear communication plan
- Make a clear and simple wound cleansing and topical care plan
- Make a clear and simple pain control plan
- Ensure that community support services are in place
- Communicate specific return and hospitalization conditions
- Set up follow-up clinic visits
- Set up long-term follow-up plans

PATIENT SELECTION

Proper patient selection is essential for out-patient care to succeed. There should be no need to monitor airway patency. The burn should be small enough, generally less than 10%, so that fluid resuscitation is not required. The patient needs to be able to drink adequate fluids (**134**). Serious burns of the face, ears, hands, genitals, or feet should generally initially be managed as in-patients (**135**). The patient's family must have the means to support an out-patient care plan. There should be an adult caregiver who can be with a young child because they may not be able to go to day care or school until healing is complete. There must be a family member, local primary care physician, or visiting nurse, who can perform wound inspections, cleansing, and dressing changes. The family must have adequate transportation so that they can come back for clinic visits and can come to the clinic or emergency department if signs of infection occur. The caregivers must be able to understand and follow the wound care and pain control plans. If there is any suspicion of abuse, out-patient management is generally contraindicated, regardless of injury severity. Finally, if it is clear on initial examination that surgery will be necessary, it is usually better to admit for prompt operation. Most patients with small burns will meet these criteria.

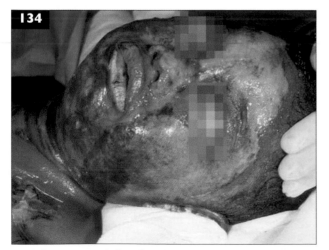

134 Patients with facial and perioral burns are often not good candidates for initial out-patient care because they may require airway monitoring and they may have trouble taking fluids by mouth.

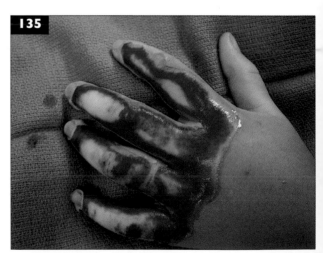

135 Significant burns of the hands or feet may not be appropriate for out-patient care, as they may require monitoring of perfusion through the period of maximal edema.

TECHNIQUES

A successful out-patient program will include teaching of the family, a clear wound cleansing and topical care plan, a clear pain control plan, utilization of community support services, a specific return and hospitalization plan, follow-up clinic visits, and long-term follow-up. A specific person should be identified to perform wound care. Wound care and dressing techniques should be demonstrated and taught, and the person to do this should verbalize their understanding.

The specific wound care plan will vary from program to program. There is a large variety of successful techniques used to care for small burns, but all share certain basics. Wounds should be periodically inspected and cleansed of accumulated exudate and desiccated topical ointments. This is done using clean rather than sterile technique, gently cleaning with clean lukewarm tap water and a bland soap. The wound should be cleansed with a gauze or clean washcloth, inspected for any sign of infection, patted dry with a clean towel, and redressed. Caregivers should be alert for wound erythema, swelling, increased tenderness, lymphangitis, odor, or drainage at the time of wound cleansing so that infectious complications can be addressed promptly. The frequency of wound cleansing and dressing change is also variable. Most small burns are adequately managed with a daily inspection, cleansing, and dressing change. This is most important in the first days after injury when most problems occur. Subsequently, less frequent dressing changes become more reasonable.

Wound dressings should prevent wound desiccation, decrease pain, reduce the incidence of wound colonization, and minimize physical trauma to the wound. Most topical agents applied in the out-patient setting have a viscous carrier that prevents wound desiccation, and a broad antibacterial spectrum that reduces wound colonization (**136**). The addition of a gauze wrap will minimize soiling of clothing and protect the wound from trauma. A brisk, calm, and gentle demeanor, with modest use of medication and liberal use of distraction, seems effective when cleaning, inspecting, and dressing small burns (**137**).

The list of available wound topicals and membranes is extensive and confusing and includes dressing materials impregnated with silver (see *Table 7*, page 24).

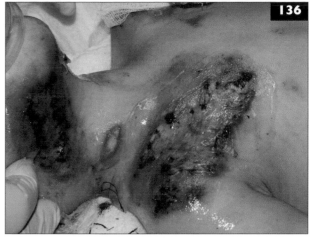

136 Wound dressings should prevent wound desiccation, decrease pain, reduce the incidence of wound colonization, and minimize physical trauma to the wound. Agents with a viscous carrier seem to minimize desiccation and reduce pain.

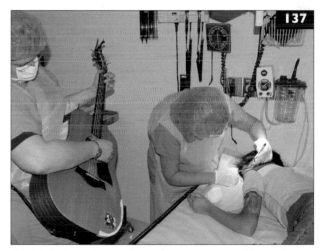

137 A brisk, calm, and gentle demeanor, with modest use of medication and liberal use of distraction, seems effective when cleaning, inspecting, and dressing small burns. Note the use of distraction to facilitate wound care in this young child.

Increasingly, membrane dressings are used in the out-patient setting, commonly after a period of topical care and daily observation (**138, 139**). There is no wrong wound dressing, as long as the above noted principles are adequately addressed. A consistent approach by all providers in a group reduces confusion.

Not every patient needs medication, but pain control should be considered in any out-patient planning. Partly occlusive wound topicals or wound membranes can greatly enhance comfort. Oftentimes, appropriate doses of acetaminophen with a narcotic given 30 min prior to a planned dressing change will suffice. Soothing children with calm speech and removing dressings slowly after thorough wetting will lessen pain and fear that can lead to failure of out-patient care. Many patients will benefit from the use of community services for transportation and visiting nurses. When available, visiting nurse services can be enormously helpful in crafting a successful out-patient program, particularly if family members do not feel capable of caring for the wound.

Regular return visits are an important component of planning. Most patients are seen at least twice weekly initially, depending on the availability of community services and the severity of the wound. At follow-up visits, wounds are cleansed and evaluated for infection and progress in healing. Developments requiring early return or hospitalization should be outlined with the patient at the time of the initial teaching. These include increased pain and anxiety that compromise wound care, inability to keep scheduled follow-up appointments, delayed healing, signs of infection, or a wound which appears deeper than initially appreciated.

Even seemingly minor burns may be the cause of intermediate-term pruritis, longer-term scarring, or other issues that may benefit from long-term burn clinic follow-up (**140**). Even if nearly perfect healing is expected, plans should be made for a visit several months after healing is complete. At that time, if there is no evidence of hypertrophic scarring, discharge to primary care follow-up is appropriate.

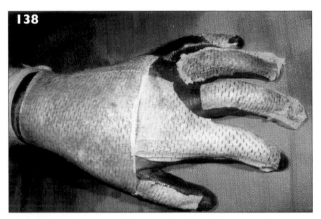

138 Porcine xenograft is applied to this wound on postinjury day 3, after a period of daily dressing change and inspection has confirmed the initial estimate of a medium depth partial-thickness burn and the absence of infection. Periodic inspection will indicate whether nonadherent portions of the membrane need replacing.

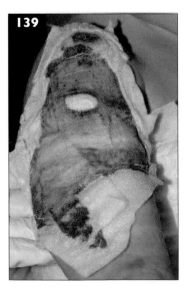

139 A silver-releasing membrane dressing has been applied to this wound. Periodic inspection will indicate the need to remove and replace saturated portions of the membrane and will exclude the development of infection.

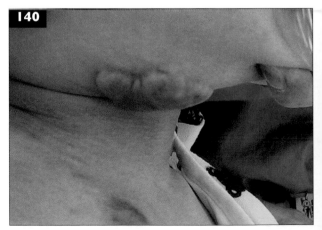

140 Even seemingly minor burns may be the cause of scarring that may benefit from long-term burn clinic follow-up.

CHAPTER 11

BURN REHABILITATION

'Don't find fault. Find a remedy.'
Henry Ford (1863–1947),
pioneering engineer and manufacturer.

'Care more for the individual patient than for the disease. The kindly word, the cheerful greeting, the sympathetic look – these the patient understands.'
Sir William Osler (1849–1919), Canadian physician.

Survival is no longer the only, or even the most important, measure of success in burn care. It has been replaced by the quality of survival. Most patients suffering serious burns are now expected to survive, and the challenge is to provide these people with high quality of function and appearance. These new standards require the intensive and ongoing involvement of interested and knowledgeable physical and occupational burn therapists. They must be part of a cohesive multidisciplinary team and their involvement must cover the entire spectrum of care, from the intensive care unit to the out-patient clinic. The relatively new field of burn therapy is rapidly evolving, filled with challenges.

EARLY ACUTE REHABILITATION

Physical and occupational therapy interventions should begin, albeit cautiously, during resuscitation of even the most serious burns, as these early interventions will facilitate later acute progress and prevent many long-term sequelae. The therapist must work closely with the critical care team so that their efforts do not interfere with immediate needs. Rehabilitation priorities in the burn intensive care unit include ranging, splinting, and antideformity positioning, and establishing short-term objectives and long-term goals with the patient and their family.

If extremities are left immobile for many days,
even in young children, capsular contraction and shortening of tendon and muscle groups crossing major joints will occur. When this happens, a predictable set of contractures will result (*Table 26*).

Table 26 Common contractures of passive positioning and prevention strategies

Neck flexion contracture:
- Daily ranging and extension splinting and conformers, split mattress (if tolerated)

Axillary adduction contracture:
- Daily ranging and abduction splinting with axillary splints or troughs

Elbow flexion and extension contractures:
- Daily ranging and alternating extension and flexion splints

Wrist flexion and extension contractures:
- Daily ranging and splinting in functional position (20° of extension)

MCP joint extension contractures:
- Daily ranging and splinting in functional position (MCP joints at 70–90° with IP joints in extension)

Hip flexion contracture:
- Daily ranging and extension splints and prone positioning (if tolerated)

Knee flexion contracture:
- Daily ranging and knee splints and knee immobilizers

Ankle extension contracture:
- Daily ranging and neutral splints

Metatarsophalangeal joint extension contractures:
- Daily ranging and splinting in functional position, rocker bottom shoes

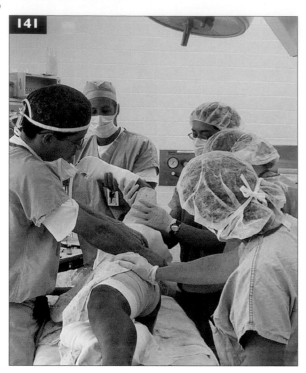

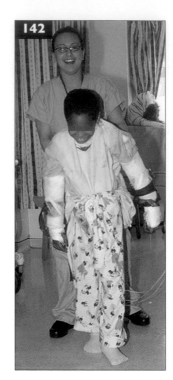

141 The therapist should be familiar with the intensive care unit and operating room, before ranging and splinting patients in these environments, so invasive devices are not misplaced or recent grafts disrupted. Here, an axillary splint is fabricated in the operating room.

142 An active and involved therapist, ranging frequently, is more effective than an isolated splinting program.

If allowed to become established, they can become very difficult to correct without additional surgery. The therapist can prevent these from occurring with regular passive ranging, splinting, and antideformity positioning. Ideally, ranging is done twice daily, with the therapist taking all joints through a passive range of motion (**141**). Some authorities believe that over-aggressive passive ranging can lead to heterotopic ossification, so this should be done with care, particularly at the elbow.

The therapist should be familiar with the complexities of the intensive care unit before doing this in critically ill patients, so invasive devices are not misplaced or recent grafts disrupted. There is substantial potential morbidity to unexpected displacement of central venous lines or endotracheal tubes, but these risks are minimal if rehabilitiation is coordinated with the critical care team. Prior to initiating ranging in critically ill patients, therapists should communicate with the intensive care unit team regarding the location and security of endotracheal tubes, nasogastric tubes, central venous catheters, arterial catheters, and other monitoring

devices. It is appropriate to medicate patients so they can tolerate the discomfort and anxiety associated with ranging as it will not be as effective if it is painful or frightening. Ideally, ranging coincides with dressing changes and wound care to take advantage of the medications given for this manipulation.

Splinting and antideformity positioning are designed to minimize facial and extremity edema and shortening of tendon and muscle groups. An active and involved therapist is more effective than an isolated splinting program (**142**). Many of these patients will be going for repetitive surgical procedures and, in consultation with the operating room team, passive ranging can be done between induction of anesthesia and preparation of the surgical site.

Troublesome contractures can be prevented by early splinting and antideformity positioning (Textbox: The relentless power of contraction, see page 98; *Table 26*). These contractures are associated with positions of comfort, except in the hands, and include neck flexion (**143, 144**), axillary adduction (**145**), elbow flexion (**146**), hip flexion (**147**), knee flexion (**148**), and ankle extension contractures (**149**).

143, 144 Neck contractures. Note how the power of contraction has deformed the mandible of the patient in (**144**).

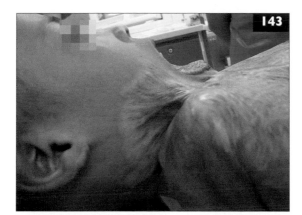

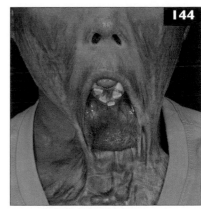

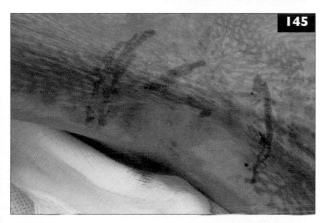

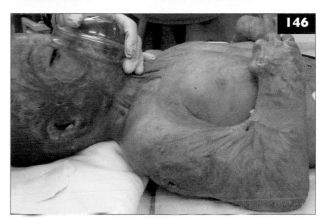

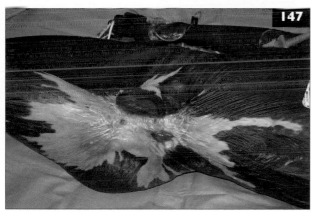

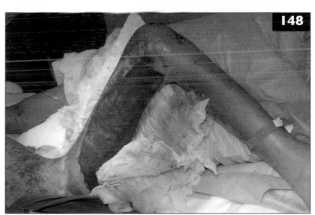

145 Modest anterior axillary adduction contracture immediately prior to correction with two incisional releases and Z-plasty. Keeping the axillary hair-bearing skin remnant in the apex of the axilla is important.

146 Elbow flexion contracture in a child with simultaneous neck and hand deformities. The prudent order of correction is neck (to facilitate airway access), then elbow (to facilitate hand positioning), followed by hand deformity correction.

147–149 Hip flexion contracture (**147**); knee flexion contracture (**148**); ankle extension contracture (**149**).

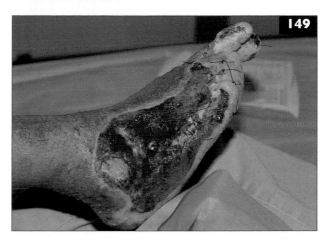

THE RELENTLESS POWER OF CONTRACTION

In 1835, Simon P. Hullihen, a 24-year-old recent graduate of the Washington College in Baltimore along with his new bride, began married life and a medical practice in Wheeling, West Virginia. One of his first referrals was the hopeless case of an unfortunate young woman with severe mandibular and facial deformities resulting from a burn years earlier. The powerful and relentless forces of contraction had deformed her teeth and mandible as well as her soft tissues. He devised an innovative (probably thought to be insane at the time) three-stage procedure which included mandibular osteotomy and correction of the soft tissue defect. He was able to perform the procedure without anesthesia, with a successful result. Many consider this the first oral surgical operation. Dr. Hullihen was perhaps the first American physician to specialize in operative dental care. In doing so, he faced the prejudice of his medical colleagues, who considered any kind of specialization suspect, and at that time, dental care was practiced by part-time mechanics. Simon Hullihen went on to perform over 1,000 oral surgical procedures, without anesthesia or antisepsis, including cleft lip and palate corrections, and mandibular reconstructions. He conceived almost all of his operations and fabricated many of his instruments, some of which are still in use. He had a reputation for kindness and frequently performed surgery for no fee. When the first college of dentistry in the United States opened in 1840, Dr. Hullihen was awarded an honorary DDS degree. His rapid rise as a national leader in dental surgery was unfortunately truncated by a fatal pneumonia at the age of 46.

Neck flexion contractures can be controlled with thermoplastic neck splints, conformers, and split mattresses. Simply positioning the neck in slight extension is often adequate. Axillary adduction can be prevented by intermittently positioning the shoulders widely abducted with axillary splints, padded hanging thermoplastic troughs, or support devices mounted to the bed (**150**). Elbow flexion and extension deformities can be minimized by statically splinting the elbow in extension, alternating with flexion splinting to facilitate a full range of motion. Hip and knee flexion contractures are especially common in infants and toddlers and will interfere with subsequent ambulation if not prevented. Prone positioning can be useful in minimizing hip flexion contractures, if patient tolerance allows. Knee immobilizers or splints can minimize knee flexion contractures (**151**).

Protracted periods of bed rest can result in prolonged periods of time with the ankle in extension. The ankle flexors will shorten and, even in the absence of an overlying burn, very troublesome equinus deformities can follow (**152**). These can be prevented with static positioning of the ankles in neutral and twice daily ranging. Once an equinus deformity is established, it can be difficult to correct with splinting, so serial casting or surgery may be required. Splints designed to position the ankle in neutral can be associated with ulceration over the metatarsal heads and calcaneus if improperly applied (**153**), particularly in heavily sedated patients. Metatarsal head pressure is prevented with local padding facilitating distribution of pressure, and pressure injuries to the heel can be prevented by extending the foot plate of the splint beyond the heel and cutting out the area around the heel. Splints should be inspected for proper fit on a regular basis to prevent progression of pressure injury to ulceration. Elevating the head and positioning

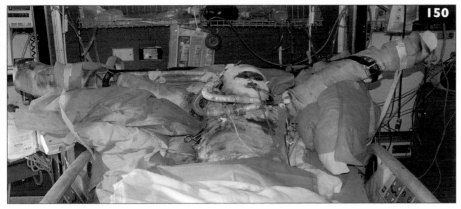

150 Padded hanging thermoplastic troughs can be used to control axillary adduction.

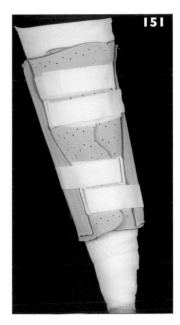

151 Knee immobilizers or splints can minimize knee flexion contractures.

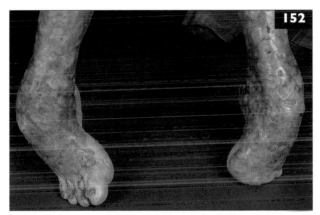

152 Ankle extension, or equinus, contractures can be minimized with static positioning of the ankles in neutral, and twice daily ranging.

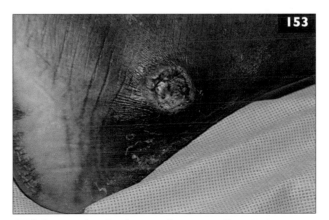

153 Proper fit of splints and wraps will minimize ulceration over bony prominences. This is a particular risk in the intensive care unit with sedated patients.

extremities above the level of the heart will minimize the facial and extremity edema associated with resuscitation (**154**).

Deep hand burns will predictably result in debilitating contractures without active intervention by burn surgeons and therapists. Although the exact contracture pattern will vary with the injury, a very common combination is hyperextension of the MCP joints, interphalangeal (IP) joint flexion, reversal of the transverse arch, web space syndactyly, and closure of the first webspace (**155**). Reconstruction of these deformities is difficult and time consuming. They are best prevented by prompt excision and closure of deep wounds with ranging and antideformity splinting.

Burn patients often need rehabilitation therapy intermittently for years. Not only is the role critical during the acute hospitalization, but there are important perioperative and scar management aftercare needs. Ideally, there is a long-term relationship between the patient and their family with the burn therapists. These relationships can enhance compliance with therapy needs and strengthen the expectation that the patient will do well and will again become active and strong. Optimistic realistic expectations greatly aid recovery.

LATE ACUTE REHABILITATION

As important as early therapeutic interventions are, they gain higher priority over other patient needs later in the acute course. In some ways, therapeutic interventions become more difficult. Patients are less sedated, more aware of what has happened to them, have been sensitized to uncomfortable procedures, and may be fearful of providers. Therapists must become part psychologist as they approach the individual's rehabilitation needs. Essential components of late acute rehabilitation include continued passive ranging, increasing active ranging, strengthening, minimizing peripheral edema, independence in activities of daily living, and preparation for work or school.

Reaching the goal of optimal function through passive and active ranging often brings some discomfort, particularly in the later acute phase of care. A balance must be found between the short-term discomfort of ranging and the long-term goal of function. An active program of passive ranging during the early phase of care pays huge dividends here. Methods useful for increasing tolerance of passive ranging include timing of ranging with medication for dressing changes, administration of NSAIDs, opiates, or benzodiazepines to facilitate therapy sessions, and gentle conversation building on the relationship formed between the patient and therapist during the early acute phase of care. Crafting therapy around enjoyed activities and play can also be very useful (**156**).

Extremity edema is common in the late acute phase of care and compromises joint mobility, particularly in the hands. Gently wrapping fingers with self-adherent elastic tapes can facilitate reduction of digital edema (**157**). Tubular elastic dressings, elastic wrap dressings, elevation, and retrograde massage will also contribute to the reduction of extremity edema. Edema is common in the feet and legs with early upright posture and ambulation. Elastic wraps when upright can reduce dependent edema and improve comfort.

As acute discharge nears, independent activities of daily living and return to work or school become the rehabilitation priorities. Resisted range of motion, isometric exercises, active strengthening, and gait training are important components. With patient and family permission, the workplace or school can be engaged in this portion of the process, smoothing the return to the community. It helps to fuel the expectation of a return to full reintegration.

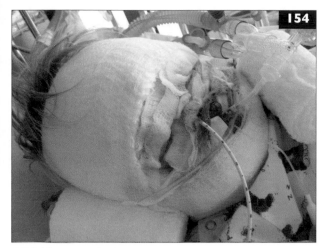

154 Elevating the head and positioning extremities above the level of the heart will minimize the facial and extremity edema associated with resuscitation.

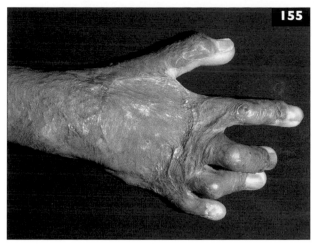

155 A common contracture combination after spontaneous healing of deep hand burns is hyperextension of the MCP joints, IP joint flexion, reversal of the transverse arch, web space syndactyly, and closure of the first webspace.

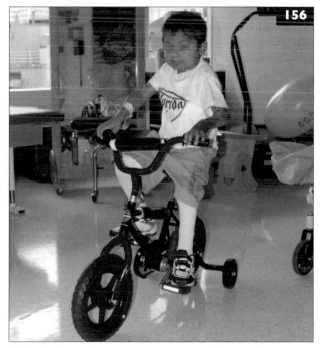

156 Crafting therapy sessions around enjoyed activities or play is very useful in late acute rehabilitation.

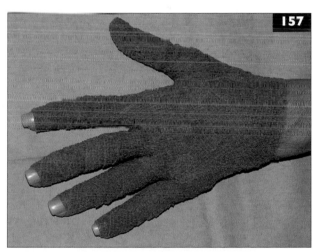

157 Hand edema is common in the late acute phase of care and compromises joint mobility. Gently wrapping fingers with self-adherent elastic tapes can facilitate reduction of digital edema.

LONG-TERM REHABILITATION AND SCAR MANAGEMENT

Burn rehabilitation bridges the transition to the outpatient environment. Important activities include progressive ranging and strengthening, evaluation of evolving problem areas, postoperative therapy after reconstructive interventions, and scar management. Ideally, the in-patient team will continue to follow the patient. This can be directly, or by periodically monitoring progress when the patient works with a general out patient therapy program closer to their home. In-patient burn therapists are an important resource for less experienced therapists assuming the care of a newly discharged burn patient. Therapists play an important role in collaborative reconstructive planning. Burn patients often have multiple reconstructive needs, and planning staged reconstruction is best done as a group, involving surgeon, family, and therapist.

Hypertrophic scar remains a difficult unsolved problem in burns (**158, 159**). All members of the team address this issue, but burn therapists generally take the lead. Typically, wound hyperemia should begin to resolve about 9 weeks after injury. In those wounds destined to become hypertrophic, neovessel formation instead increases, resulting in increasing erythema and subsequent contraction and hypertrophy. Although the physiology of hypertrophic scarring remains an enigma, its clinical consequences are well known, and many useful interventions have been demonstrated.

Established interventions include scar massage, compression garments, topical silicone, steroid injections, and surgery. Serial casting may help selected functionally limiting hypertrophic scars that cross major joints. When frequently and properly performed, scar massage is quite effective and can be done by patients and family members. Firm massage and stretching of evolving hypertrophic areas after application of bland ointments is ideally done several times each day. Compression garments are expensive and uncomfortable, but there is substantial anecdotal evidence that they do facilitate control of broad areas of hypertrophic scarring, especially in young children, in whom hypertrophic scarring seems to be especially severe. To achieve optimal effect, compression garments are worn for the bulk of each day until wound erythema begins to abate 12–18 months after injury. In growing children they need frequent refitting and replacement. Compression masks, molded by hand or custom fabricated with a helium–neon laser-

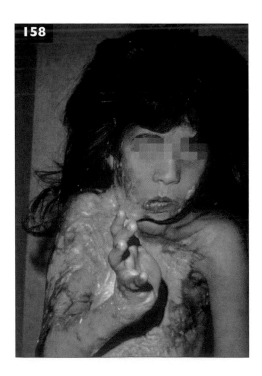

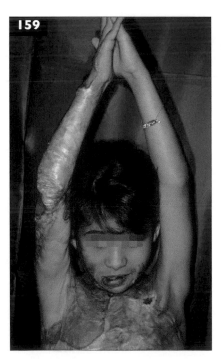

158, 159 Hypertrophic scar remains a very difficult unsolved problem in burns.

derived digital map, can be effective adjuncts to management of facial scars (**160**). Topical silicone sheets seem effective when applied to small areas of troublesome hypertrophic scar. Rashes often occur beneath the topical silicone, but usually quickly resolve with removal and briefer periods of application.

Localized early hypertrophic scars in important aesthetic cosmetic locations or which cause significant localized pruritus often respond favorably to 1–3 steroid injections spaced over several weeks. Injecting dense scars is painful and requires anesthesia in children. Surgical incision or excision, release, and grafting are very important components of scar management. Hypertrophic scars seem to enlarge when there is local tension, and diffuse regional reduction of scar thickness often follows the local release of tension associated with surgery. Z-plasties are also very effective in reducing local tension and thereby scar thickness (**161, 162**). Steroid injections can also be a useful adjunct in very localized evolving hypertrophic scars. They can reduce localized pruritis.

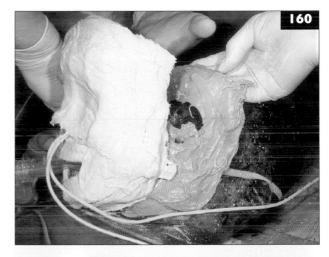

160 Compression masks, molded by hand or custom fabricated with a helium–neon laser-derived digital map, can be effective adjuncts to management of facial scars.

161, 162 Diffuse regional reduction of scar thickness often follows the local release of tension associated with incisional release and/or Z-plasties. (Courtesy of Dr. Mathias B. Donelan.)

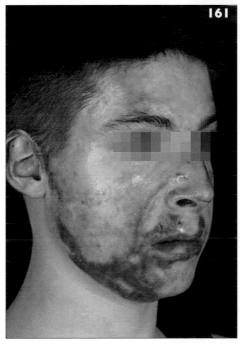

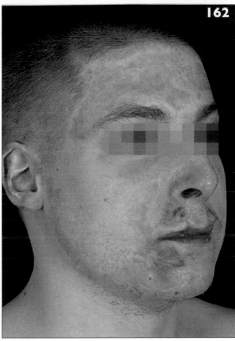

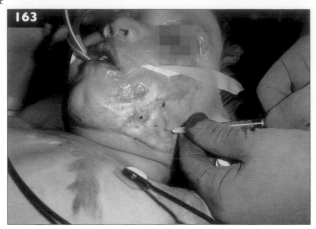

163 Steroid injections can be a useful adjunct in very localized evolving hypertrophic scars. They can be used to reduce localized pruritis. However, overuse can contribute to telangiectasia.

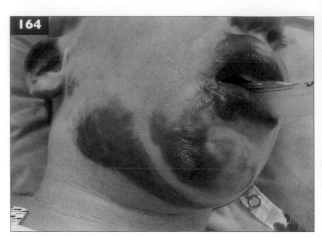

164 Tuneable dye laser treatments are being trialled as an adjunct to reduce wound hypertrophy, the concept being that it will limit early neovessel formation. This is not currently part of the standard of care as a stand-alone treatment.

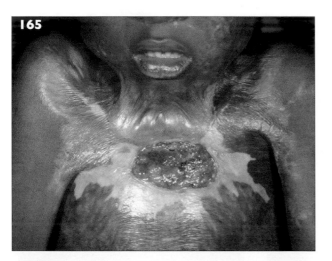

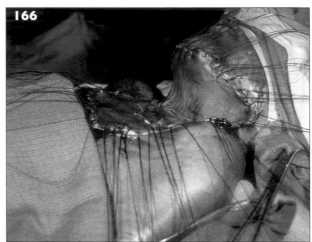

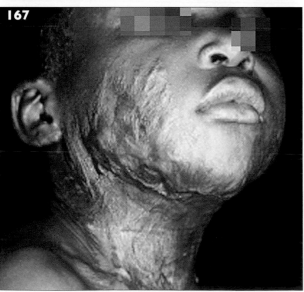

165–167 In some patients, ulcerations within hypertrophic scars will become chronic and recurrent, usually caused by local tension. In most of these, durable healing can be achieved by local release and grafting.

168, 169 Rarely, a chronic ulceration in a burn wound will develop into a squamous cell cancer. Chronic ulcers should be excised and sent for histologic examination, or followed closely with biopsy, as these cancers can be aggressive.

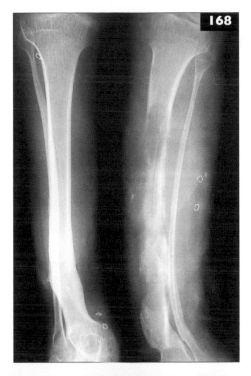

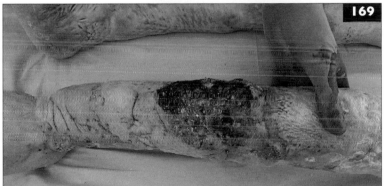

However, overuse can contribute to telangiectasia (**163**). Tuneable dye laser treatments are being trialled as an adjunct to reduce wound hypertrophy, the concept being that it will limit early neovessel formation (**164**). At present, it cannot be recommended as the standard of care.

Many late acute burn patients are bothered by pruritus. This usually begins shortly after the wound is healed, peaks 4–6 months after injury, and then gradually subsides in most patients. It can be especially difficult at night. When bothersome, it is usually adequately managed with massage, and bedtime oral antihistamines. Many other remedies exist, although none reliably works in everyone. If patients are particularly troubled by pruritus, therapeutic trials may identify one which is particularly helpful for that individual. These include scratching or slapping overlying compression garments, topical vitamin E, topical antihistamines, topical cold compresses, moisturizing creams, and colloidal baths. Localized highly pruritic scars will often respond nicely to a steroid injection. In most patients, this difficult issue can be worked through, as wounds mature and pruritis abates.

In some patients, ulcerations within hypertrophic scars will become chronic and recurrent. This situation is most commonly caused by local tension. Quite often, durable healing can be achieved by release and grafting (**165–167**). Rarely, a chronic ulceration in a burn wound will develop into a squamous cell cancer (**168, 169**). Older chronic ulcers should be excised and sent for histologic examination, or followed closely with biopsy, as these cancers can be aggressive.

AUSTERE ALTERNATIVES: BURN REHABILITATION

In many developing environments, burn rehabilitation is severely limited by inadequate numbers of practitioners, inadequate funding, and inadequate transportation. Compromises will be necessary. Family involvement and teaching may be used to good effect in many situations. Outside funding can be used to develop low-cost and highly effective programs, but these will be limited. In the absence of therapists and compression garments, families can be taught how to range joints and provide scar massage, both of which are highly effective when consistently applied (**170**).

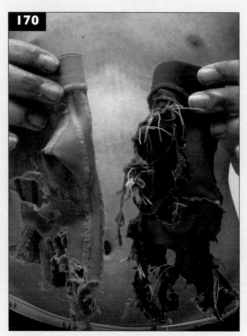

170 Compression garments are often impractical or unavailable. They may become worn, as shown here, and not be replaceable. Fortunately, scar massage can be very effective when practiced by trained family members.

Chapter 12

Acute Burn Reconstruction and Aftercare

'A journey of a thousand miles begins with a single step.'
Confucius (551–479 BCE),
teacher, scholar, philosopher.

'People will forget what you said, people will forget what you did, but people will never forget how you made them feel.'
Maya Angelou (1928–present), American poet.

Depending on patient desire, injury severity, and resource availability, staged burn reconstruction can be unnecessary or last a lifetime. There is a core set of early reconstructive operations commonly required during the first years after injury (Textbox: What is burn surgery?). If these needs are met, patients reach independent function earlier and later reconstructive efforts can more effectively provide them high-quality functional and aesthetic results they have every right to expect. These needs are optimally delivered by the acute care team as the procedures often overlap late acute burn and wound priorities, and the relationship between this team and the patient is well established. An acute reconstructive plan should be made collaboratively with the patient and their family, the patient's therapists, and the surgical team. These operations are generally very well tolerated. Waiting for complete scar maturation in the face of obvious functional needs interferes with recovery.

WHAT IS BURN SURGERY?

In the years before the First World War, burn patients were cared for principally by medical physicians. As surgical options grew, burn patients came under the care of general surgeons. As the field of plastic surgery blossomed, particularly after the Second World War, plastic surgery programs took on these tasks. With the development of acute excisional burn operations, and their supporting surgical critical care and resuscitation needs, general and trauma surgeons began increasingly to manage burn units. As the field now stands, burn patients need the surgical skills of general, trauma, pediatric, and plastic surgeons. They need skilled surgical intensivists. Burn surgery has evolved to be a field half-way between trauma and plastic surgery. Practitioners of burn surgery need to bring all of these skills to their patients, as individuals or as part of a seamless collaboration. In North America, most burn surgeons arrive via the trauma/general surgery training track. In Europe, most arrive via the plastic surgery track. Without further training or experience, neither training package alone is generally adequate to practice burn surgery at a high level. The American Burn Association has recently published criteria for fellowship training in burn surgery, which includes critical care certification and elements of general, trauma, plastic, and pediatric surgery. Increasingly, burn surgeons arrive via this common fellowship pathway, whatever their initial training.

HEAD AND NECK

Soft tissues of the face are very compliant and easily distorted by the forces of contraction. The focus of early acute facial reconstruction should be primarily functional, keeping in mind techniques that will optimize appearance as well. Reconstructive needs can be minimized by initial resurfacing with thick sheet grafts and early attention to scar management. However, even in the best of circumstances, a limited number of stereotypical facial deformities are common and should be addressed early. Common early postacute facial reconstructive needs include eyelid ectropion, lip eversion, microstomia, thickened nasolabial bands, medial canthal webs, and neck contracture. These are all amenable to relatively simple corrective procedures that can make a huge difference to facial function and patient self-esteem.

Eyelid ectropion occur because the lids are so compliant that adjacent contractile forces will expose the globe (see **76, 77**). Corrective procedures are commonly needed by patients with periocular burns during acute care. A need for one or more revisions is not at all uncommon. In most cases, the normal lid remnant can be unrolled superficially, retaining normal lid function. If deeper incisions violate the orbital septum, unsightly protrusion of periorbital fat may occur. If the tarsal plate is devascularized or perforated, coverage of the globe can be threatened. Tarsorrhaphy is rarely needed, as well designed tie-over bolsters will provide graft fixation and stability while retaining some ability to see in the immediate postoperative period (**171, 172**).

Despite prompt grafting with thick sheet grafts and good wound care, deep burns of the submental area and neck are frequently followed by contracture formation. When neck contractures are functionally important or cause chronic neck discomfort, neck release is indicated. This is especially important if access to the airway is compromised (**173–175**). Most patients obtain excellent results with incisional release and split-thickness autografting. Some contractures of limited extent are amenable to Z-plasty revision (**176**). The compliant tissues of the neck and mobility of the head make fairly extreme deformity common (**177**). The surgeon should be in the operating room on induction of anesthesia in such cases, as urgent neck or commisure release may be needed. Long-term results are better if patients can be compliant with splinting programs. Even so, the compliant tissues of this region make revision common.

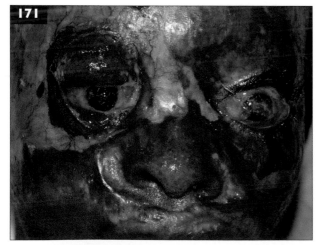 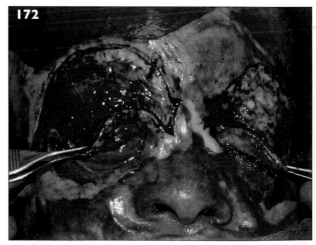

171, 172 Even in severe ectropia, as seen here, the normal lid remnant can usually be unrolled superficially, retaining normal lid function. Tarsorrhaphy is rarely needed, as well designed tie-over bolsters will provide graft fixation and stability while retaining some ability to see in the immediate postoperative period.

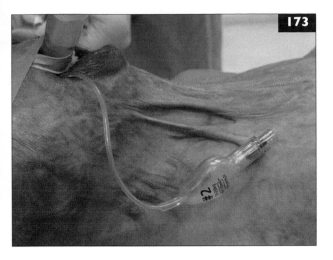

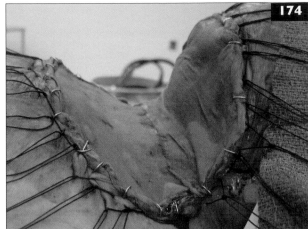

173–175 When neck contractures are functionally important or cause chronic neck discomfort, neck release is indicated. Most patients obtain excellent results with incisional release and split-thickness autografting. In some cases (**175**), combined release of the neck, torso, and axillae is required.

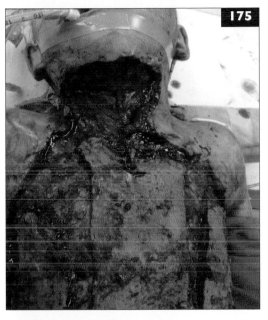

176 Some contractures of limited extent are amenable to Z-plasty revision.

177 If neck contracture compromises access to the airway, the surgeon should be in the operating room on induction of anesthesia in case urgent neck or commisure release is needed.

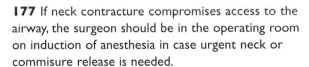

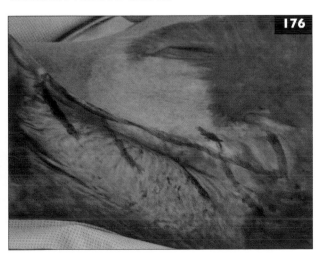

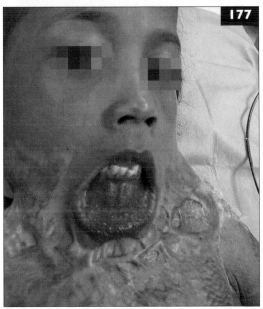

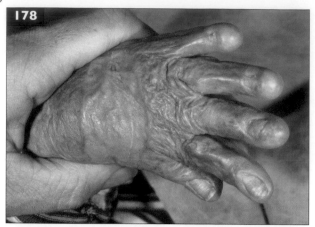

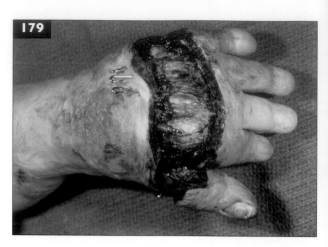

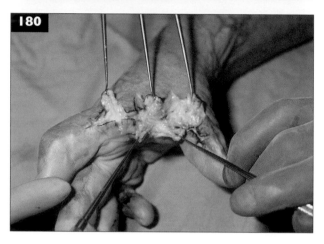

178, 179 When needed, dorsal release should be performed proximal to the MCP joints. The goal of the release is to achieve a resistance-free complete range of motion of the MCP joints. In some cases, temporary axial Kirschner wires are useful to hold position, but are removed within 2–3 weeks.

180 Modest webspace contractures can sometimes be corrected with 5-flap Z-plasties.

HAND

The highly mobile nature of the hand makes it prone to the inexorable forces of wound contraction. The most common hand deformities requiring early correction depend on injury pattern in individual patients, but include MCP extension or 'dorsal hand' contractures, interdigital and first web space contractures, palmar contractures, and IP flexion contractures. A particularly difficult form of the latter is the 'burn boutonnière' deformity. The weak extensors of the fifth finger make it particularly prone to flexion contracture. Many hand contractures can be prevented by early grafting of full-thickness burns followed by attentive therapy. However, in the growing hands of young children, many of these deformities cannot be prevented and revisions are a necessary fact of life.

MCP extension or dorsal hand contratures are ideally prevented by grafting of full-thickness dorsal hand burns followed by proper positioning, splinting, and therapy. When needed, dorsal release should be done proximal to the MCP joints (**178, 179**). The goal of the release is to achieve a resistance-free complete range of motion of the MCP joints. In some cases, temporary axial Kirschner wires are useful to hold position, but are removed within 2–3 weeks.

Interdigital and first web space contractures, or 'burn syndactyly' are more commonly dorsal, but they can be volar or mixed in location. In the normal web space, the trailing dorsal edge of the webspace slopes at a gentle 45° to the leading volar edge. Minor webspace contractures do not interfere with function, but as they advance they will interfere with abduction of the digits and this should be addressed. Modest deformities can sometimes be corrected with 5-flap Z-plasties (**180**). More advanced deformities usually require release and full- or thick split-thickness autografting. Dorsal or volar wrist contractures generally respond well to incisional release and grafting (**181–184**).

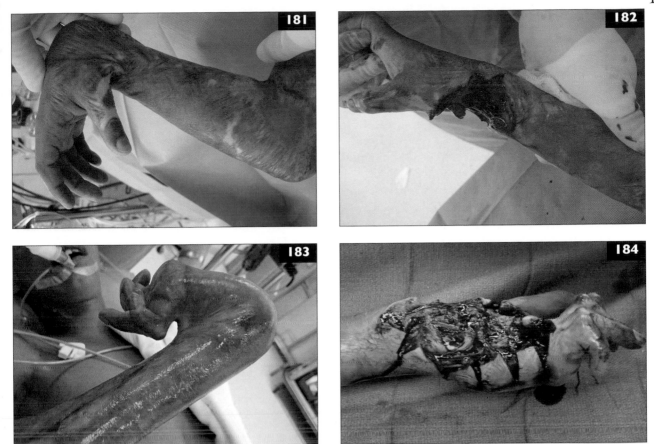

181–184 Dorsal or volar wrist contractures generally respond well to incisional release and grafting. These are ideally addressed before, or simultaneously with, finger deformity correction.

Palmar contractures are especially common in growing young children, even when their burns have been very well managed. Surgery can often be delayed until there is some interference with function to minimize the number of interventions over the years of growth, but needing repeated operations is not uncommon. These defects usually respond very well to stellate incisional release and full-thickness grafting (**185**).

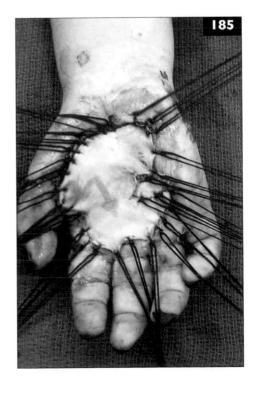

185 Palmar contractures are generally well managed with stellate incisional release and full-thickness grafting.

Patients with darker skin tones are sometimes managed with split-thickness plantar grafts harvested from the sole of the foot to avoid pigment mismatch (**186**), but donor site morbidity may not justify this in every case.

IP flexion contractures of the digits are common. When relatively minor, they will respond nicely to Z-plasty revision (**187**, **188**). When more advanced, incisional release and full-thickness grafting are required. More difficult are burn boutonnière fifth finger deformities. The burn boutonnière describes the situation where the extensor mechanism has been so damaged that the lateral bands slip volar, and become IP joint flexors (**189**, **190**). This is very often associated with an open IP joint and is usually impossible to reconstruct. Sometimes, when performed early, volar release and grafting with axial wire fixation and subsequent extensor splinting will suffice. More often, simultaneous arthrodesis is required. The deeply burned fifth finger is very prone to severe flexion deformity, especially in young children who are hard to splint. These can be addressed with release, full- or thick split-thickness grafting, and axial wire fixation with generally very good results. Occasional patients will require arthrodesis. Rarely, repair of the dorsal extensor apparatus is possible (**191**). In most of these procedures, tie-over bolsters provide excellent graft stabilization, but distal digital perfusion should be verified before emergence from anesthesia.

UPPER EXTREMITY

Recovering patients need a functional range of elbow motion to perform activities of daily living, such as eating and toileting. Patients with deep upper extremity burns not infrequently develop elbow contractures in flexion, with an inability to extend. These are fairly easy to improve with soft tissue release and graft, often supplemented with Z-plasties (**192**, **193**). Soft tissue contractures with limited ability to flex are much less common, but similarly managed.

Heterotopic ossification about the elbow develops in many patients with particularly deep burns in this area. For unclear reasons, these patients develop soft tissue ossification in the triceps tendon and pericapsular soft tissues. Initially, they usually have excessive pain with movement. At this early stage, plain radiographs are often normal, but more sensitive

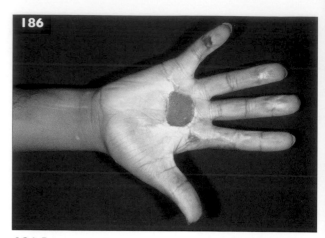

186 Patients with darker skin tones are sometimes managed with split-thickness plantar grafts harvested from the sole of the foot to avoid the pigment mismatch seen here, but donor site morbidity may not justify this in many cases.

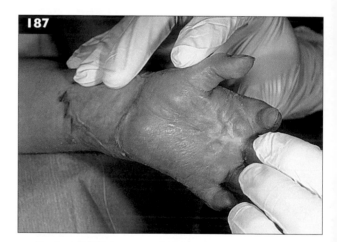

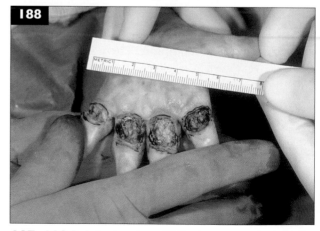

187, 188 Relatively minor IP flexion contractures of the digits respond nicely to Z-plasty revision. When more advanced, incisional release and full-thickness grafting are required.

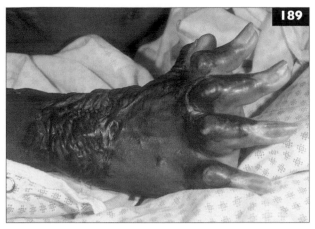

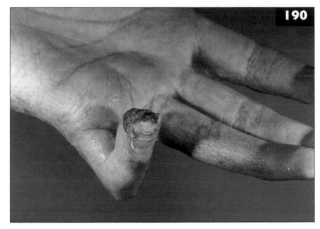

189, 190 The burn boutonnière describes the situation where the extensor mechanism has been so damaged that the lateral bands slip volar, and become IP joint flexors. This is often associated with an open IP joint and is usually impossible to reconstruct. Sometimes, when done early, volar release and grafting with axial wire fixation and subsequent extensor splinting will suffice. More often, simultaneous arthrodesis is required for established deformities.

191 The deeply burned fifth finger is prone to severe flexion deformity, especially in young children who are hard to splint. These can be addressed with release, full- or thick split thickness grafting, and axial wire fixation with generally very good results in most patients. Occasionally, arthrodesis is required. Rarely, repair of the dorsal extensors is possible. (Courtesy of Dr. Jonathon Winograd.)

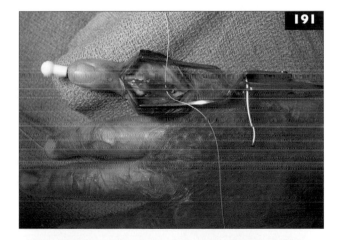

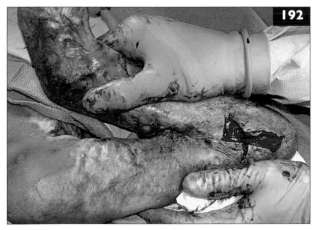

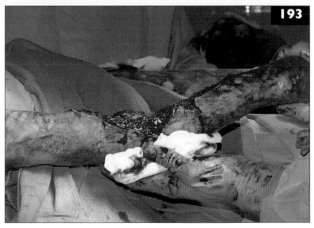

192, 193 Most elbow contractures are fairly easy to improve with soft tissue release and graft supplemented with Z-plasties. Soft tissue contractures with limited ability to flex are much less common, but similarly managed. Combined upper extremity contractures are best managed proximal to distal in sequential or combined operations.

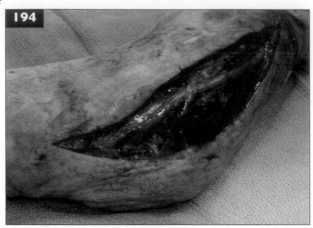

194 Heterotopic ossification can be improved when overlying grafts are durably healed via axial incision. Heterotopic bone is removed enough to improve motion. The ulnar nerve should be protected and may need to be transposed. These elbows are typically deeply burned and perioperative wound problems are common, but long-term results are often excellent.

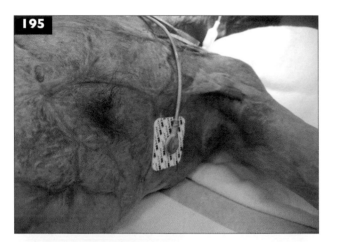

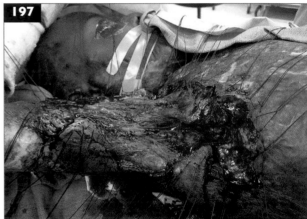

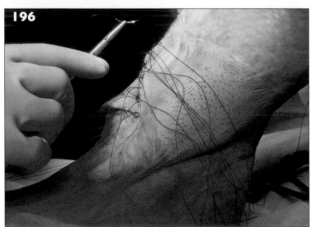

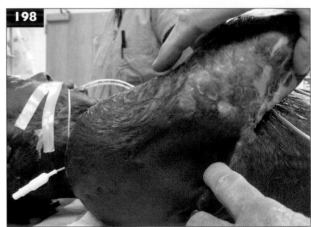

195, 196 Poorly planned releases can move remnant axillary hair-bearing skin to ectopic locations. In these two cases, multiple prior releases have moved the remnant onto the chest wall or the arm. This is a particular risk in prepubescent children, but can usually be prevented by thoughtful operative planning.

197, 198 Keeping any axillary hair-bearing skin remnant in the apex of the axilla can be done through careful operative planning. In many cases, incisional releases above and below the axilla allow any remnant to collapse up into the apex of the axilla.

studies, such as CT scanning, may demonstrate heterotopic bone formation (see **82**). This may resolve on its own over the course of months, but when it becomes severe, it rarely resolves. In severe cases, decreasing range is rapid, and can progress to functional fusion. In these patients, the rehabilitation priority should become the maintenance of functional range of motion, rather than complete range. In patients with severe bilateral heterotopic ossification, this means that one elbow (usually the one with the better hand) should be allowed to fuse functionally in flexion, to be useful in feeding, and the other should be allowed to fuse functionally in extension, to be useful in toileting. When overlying grafts are durably healed, the elbow can be approached from a posterior axial incision and the heterotopic bone removed enough to improve motion (**194**). The ulnar nerve should be protected and may need to be transposed. These elbows are typically deeply burned and perioperative wound problems are common, but long-term results are often excellent.

Axillary contracture is not uncommon during the early recovery period in patients with upper body burns. A tight axillary contracture can interfere with activities of daily living and with play. Axillary releases should encompass the entire axis of rotation of the shoulder to facilitate complete range of motion in all planes. It is important to ensure that any remnant of axillary hair-bearing skin remains in the apex of the axilla. Poorly planned releases can move this remnant, when present, to ectopic locations (**195, 196**), or even split it. In many cases, incisional releases above and below the axilla allow this remnant to collapse up into the apex of the axilla (**197, 198**). Most axillary contractures are not completely correctable with Z-plasty, but Z-plasty is often useful to enhance results obtained with stellate release and graft (**199**). Rotation flaps are occasionally useful in modest contractures. Post-operative abduction splints can help retain range but should not cause traction or pressure on the brachial plexus.

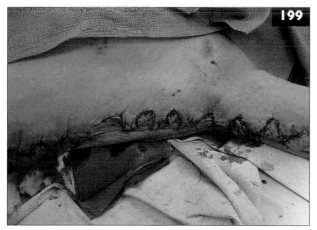

199 Most axillary contractures are not completely correctable with Z-plasty, but they are often useful to enhance results obtained with stellate release and graft.

LOWER EXTREMITY

Common early contractures seen in patients recovering from deep lower extremity burns include metatarsophalangeal (MTP) joint extension contractures (dorsal forefoot contractures), interdigital webbing and IP joint flexion contractures of the toes, popliteal flexion contractures, hip and groin flexion contractures, and perineal contractures. A combination of hip and popliteal flexion contractures is particularly common in infants, who tend to spend long periods of time with the hips and knees flexed and who are difficult to splint and range.

The dorsal forefoot contracture (MTP joint extension contracture) is common in patients with deep dorsal foot burns, particularly growing young children. They can develop compromised ambulation when unable to touch toes to the floor. They respond readily to dorsal release and graft, occasionally requiring temporary axial wire fixation (**200, 201**). Interdigital webbing (burn syndactyly) is much less often symptomatic in the toes when compared to the hands, but is well managed in a similar fashion (**202**).

Popliteal flexion contractures are particularly common in infants and children and can interfere with ambulation. These are generally straightforward operations responding to stellate transverse release and sheet grafting. It is important to avoid injury to the relatively superficial neurovascular structures of the popliteal fossa and peroneal nerve at the knee. Flexion contractures of the hip and groin are also especially common in infants and young children, also compromising ambulation. Results with stellate release and sheet grafting are reliably good (**203, 204**). It is important to be sensitive to the location of the femoral vessels and nerve during these operations, as the overlying contracted tissues may distort normal anatomy.

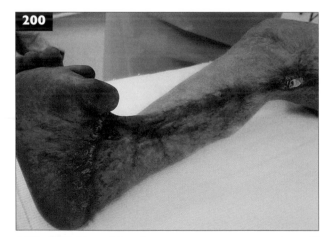
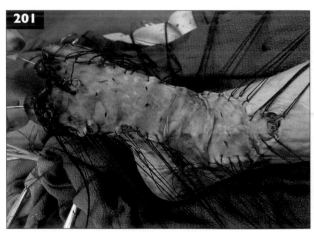

200, 201 Dorsal forefoot contractures respond readily to dorsal release and graft, occasionally requiring temporary axial wire fixation and simultaneous webspace releases.

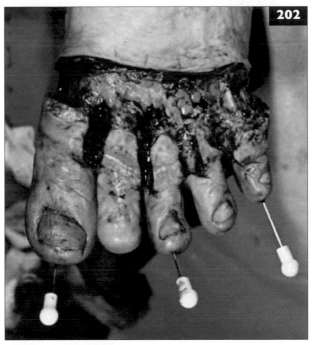

202 Syndactyly of the toes is much less symptomatic than that of the fingers, but can be similarly managed.

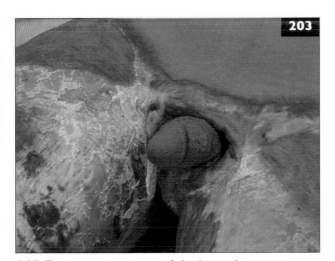

203 Flexion contractures of the hip and groin can interfere with ambulation and upright posture. They seem especially common in infants and young children. Stellate release and sheet grafting are generally very successful.

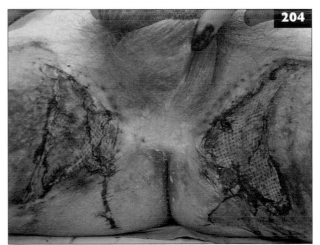

204 Perineal bands are best corrected with paired lateral releases.

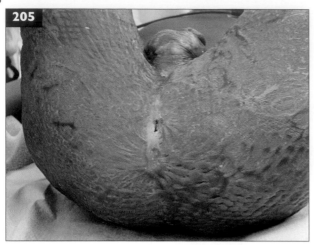

205 Some patients with deep perianal burns will develop quite symptomatic contractures that interfere with defecation, and even ambulation. These can be approached with stellate release and grafting with generally good results. Protection of the sphincter mechanism is important.

THE GUINEA PIG CLUB

Dr. Sir Archibald McIndoe (1900–1960) was born in Dunedin, New Zealand, into a middle class family, studying medicine at the University of Otago, pathology at the Mayo Clinic, and surgery in London under his cousin, plastic surgeon Harold Gillies. He subsequently worked in London as a general and then plastic surgeon. After the outbreak of the Second World War, he was appointed consultant in plastic surgery to the Royal Air Force, and was assigned to the Queen Victoria Hospital in East Grinstead, West Sussex. Through the war years, he was faced with airmen who had survived disfiguring burns, and who faced lives of isolation. McIndoe changed the treatment paradigm. He was both an innovative technician and a compassionate human being. He developed novel techniques for treating severe facial and hand deformities. Most remarkable for his time, he perceived the importance of emotional recovery. During long staged reconstructions, his team facilitated the social recovery and reintegration of his patients. Over 600 burned flyers underwent staged innovative operations at East Grinstead. Many of the operations were new and untried, so the patients proclaimed themselves members of the 'Guinea Pig Club' (**206**). After the war he received many awards, being knighted in 1947, as much for his restoration of the minds of his patients as their bodies. He died in 1960, after a distinguished career in academic plastic surgery.

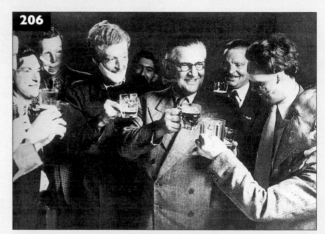

206 Sir Archibald McIndoe's results were spectacular. He healed his patients physically and also understood the importance of emotional healing and of belonging to a group. Similar principles are followed today by burn recovery groups, such as the Phoenix Society. (Reproduced by kind permission of the author and publisher from *The Reconstruction of Warriors: Archibald McIndoe, the Royal Air Force and the Guinea Pig Club* by E.R. Mayhew. Greenhill Books, London, 2004.)

Some patients with perineal burns will develop a transverse band across the perineum that becomes quite symptomatic, interfering with ambulation, sexual function, and defecation. They can be effectively approached with a stellate incisional release high on each medial thigh, allowing the band to fall back into the apex of the perineum. Some patients with deep perianal burns will develop quite symptomatic contractures that interfere with defecation, and even ambulation. These can be approached with stellate release and grafting with generally good results (**205**). Protection of the sphincter mechanism is important.

AFTERCARE AND EMOTIONAL RECOVERY

Ultimately, our success as burn care providers is judged by the success of our patients in their efforts to reintegrate with their communities and families (Textbox: The Guinea Pig Club). These successes cannot occur without excellent acute care and reconstruction, but there is increasing evidence demonstrating that ongoing participation in a coordinated burn aftercare program enhances outcomes. Increasingly, burn aftercare programs are important components of burn centers.

A coordinated burn aftercare program includes ready access to an out-patient burn clinic, social work support, psychologic and psychiatric assistance, as well as surgical and nursing care. Identification and treatment of those suffering from post-traumatic stress facilitate recovery. In many programs, burn survivor peer support has been found useful to facilitate successful reintegration. A particularly successful program is sponsored by the Phoenix Society for Burn Survivors.

The tools and techniques we can bring to our patients are far better than they were 30 years ago. To achieve the outcomes we want requires a devoted effort by the burn team over years. For many of our patients and their families, the burn will be the most traumatic event of their life. It is a great privilege to participate in their recovery.

AUSTERE ALTERNATIVES

Even when initial care has been flawless and rehabilitation therapy conscientiously applied, burn reconstruction is often necessary to ensure optimal functional and aesthetic results. Further, many patients will benefit from psychologic support to enjoy a full emotional recovery. In the developing world, reconstruction and aftercare services are limited severely by funding realities. The resulting functional disabilities and cosmetic deformities greatly compromise the lives of burn survivors. In some settings, partnerships with burn programs in the developed world can lead to some improvement, with reconstructive surgery provided by visiting teams, such as Interplast or Physicians for Peace. Optimally, government and charitable programs can be developed. The unmet long-term needs of burn patients, particularly for reconstruction, remain a pressing reality in many parts of the world.

SELECTED READING

CHAPTER 1
RECENT HISTORY

Burke JF, Quinby WC, Jr., Bondoc CC. Primary excision and prompt grafting as routine therapy for the treatment of thermal burns in children. 1976 [classical article]. *Hand Clinics* 1990;**6**:305–17.

Herndon DN, Gore D, Cole M, *et al*. Determinants of mortality in pediatric patients with greater than 70% full-thickness total body surface area thermal injury treated by early total excision and grafting. *J Trauma* 1987;**27**:208–12.

Janzekovic Z. A new concept in the early excision and immediate grafting of burns. *J Trauma* 1970;**10**:1103–8.

Saffle JR. The 1942 fire at Boston's Cocoanut Grove nightclub. *Am J Surg* 1993;**166**:581–91.

EPIDEMIOLOGY

Brigham PA, McLoughlin E. Burn incidence and medical care use in the United States: estimates, trends, and data sources. *J Burn Care Rehabil* 1996;**17**:95–107.

Derrett S, Davie G, Ameratunga S, Langley J. Capturing outcomes following injury: a New Zealand pilot study. *N Z Med J* 2010;**123**(1316):66–74.

Erdmann TC, Feldman KW, Rivara FP, Heimbach DM, Wall HA. Tap water burn prevention: the effect of legislation. *Pediatrics* 1991;**88**:572–7.

Sellar C, Ferguson JA, Goldacre MJ. Occurrence and repetition of hospital admissions for accidents in preschool children. *BMJ* 1991;**302**:16–9.

Sheridan RL, Ryan CM, Petras LM, Lydon MK, Weber JM, Tompkins RG. Burns in children younger than two years of age: an experience with 200 consecutive admissions. *Pediatrics* 1997;**100**:721–3.

ORGANIZATION OF BURN CARE

American College of Surgeons: Committee on Trauma. *Resources of Optimal Care of the Injured Patient*. Chicago: American College of Surgeons, 2006.

Mullins RJ, Veum-Stone J, Hedges JR, *et al*. Influence of a statewide trauma system on location of hospitalization and outcome of injured patients. *J Trauma* 1996;**40**:536–45; discussion 545–6.

Sheridan RL. The evolution of burn centers and burn care systems. In: Saffle J (ed). *Thermal Injuries. Problems in General Surgery* 2003;**20**(1):1–6.

Sheridan R, Weber J, Prelack K, Petras L, Lydon M, Tompkins R. Early burn center transfer shortens the length of hospitalization and reduces complications in children with serious burn injuries. *J Burn Care Rehabil* 1999;**20**:347–50.

LONG-TERM OUTCOMES

Kucan J, Bryant E, Dimick A, Sundance P, Cope N, Richards R, Anderson C. Systematic care management: a comprehensive approach to catastrophic injury management applied to a catastrophic burn injury population: clinical, utilization, economic and outcome data in support of the model. *J Burn Care Res* 2010;**31**(5):692–700.

Moore P, Blakeney P, Broemeling L, Portman S, Herndon DN, Robson M. Psychologic adjustment after childhood burn injuries as predicted by personality traits [see comments]. *J Burn Care Rehabil* 1993;**14**:80–2.

Sheridan RL, Hinson MI, Liang MH, *et al*. Long-term outcome of children surviving massive burns. *JAMA* 2000;**283**:69–73.

CHAPTER 2
LOCAL RESPONSE TO BURN INJURY

Aggarwal SJ, Diller KR, Blake GK, Baxter CR. Burn-induced alterations in vasoactive function of the peripheral cutaneous microcirculation. *J Burn Care Rehabil* 1994;**15**:1–12.

Mooney EK. Daniel Drake's account of his own hand burns (1830). *Plast Reconstr Surg* 1998;**102**:1748–54.

SYSTEMIC RESPONSE TO BURN INJURY

Dahiya P. Burns as a model of SIRS. *Front Biosci* 2009;**14**:4962–7.

Pereira CT, Herndon DN. The pharmacologic modulation of the hypermetabolic response to burns. *Adv Surg* 2005;**39**:245–61.

Sasaki TM, Welch GW, Herndon DN, Kaplan JZ, Lindberg RB, Pruitt BA, Jr. Burn wound manipulation-induced bacteremia. *J Trauma* 1979;**19**:46–8.

PEDIATRIC CONSIDERATIONS

Fabia R, Groner JI. Advances in the care of children with burns. *Adv Pediatr* 2009;**56**:219–48.

Graves TA, Cioffi WG, McManus WF, Mason AD, Jr., Pruitt BA, Jr. Fluid resuscitation of infants and children with massive thermal injury. *J Trauma* 1988;**28**:1656–9.

McManus WF, Hunt JL, Pruitt BA, Jr. Postburn convulsive disorders in children. *J Trauma* 1974;**14**:396–401.

Sheridan RL, Remensnyder JP. Management of the seriously burned infant. *J Burn Care Rehabil* 1998;**19**(2):115–8.

GERIATRIC CONSIDERATIONS

Khadim MF, Rashid A, Fogarty B, Khan K. Mortality estimates in the elderly burn patients: The Northern Ireland experience. *Burns* 2009;**35**(1):107–13.

McGill V, Kowal-Vern A, Gamelli RL. Outcome for older burn patients. *Arch Surg* 2000;**135**(3):320–5.

Ryan CM, Schoenfeld DA, Thorpe WP, Sheridan RL, Cassem EH, Tompkins RG. Objective estimates of the probability of death from burn injuries. *N Engl J Med* 1998;**338**:362–6.

Sheridan RL, Prelack K, Yin L. Energy needs are poorly predicted in critically ill elderly. *J Intensive Care Med* 1997;**12**:45–9.

CHAPTER 3
PREHOSPITAL AND INTERHOSPITAL TRANSPORT
Cochran A, Edelman LS, Morris SE, Saffle JR. Learner satisfaction with Web-based learning as an adjunct to clinical experience in burn surgery. *J Burn Care Res* 2008;**29**(1):222–6.

Renz EM, Cancio LC, Barillo DJ, *et al*. Long range transport of war-related burn casualties. *J Trauma* 2008;**64**(2 Suppl):S136–44.

Sheridan RL, Prelack K, Lydon M, Petras L, Tompkins RG. Implications of delayed transfer of seriously burned children. *J Burn Care Rehabil* 1999;**20**(5):347–50.

PRIMARY SURVEY
Helvig B, Mlcak R, Nichols RJ, Jr. Anchoring endotracheal tubes on patients with facial burns. Review from Shriners Burns Institute, Galveston, Texas. *J Burn Care Rehabil* 1987;**8**:236–7.

Sheridan RL. Recognition and management of hot liquid aspiration in children. *Ann Emerg Med* 1996;**27**:89–91.

SECONDARY SURVEY
Sheridan RL, Shank ES. Hyperbaric oxygen treatment: a brief overview of a controversial topic. *J Trauma* 1999;**47**:426–35.

Wachtel TL. Epidemiology, classification, initial care, and administrative considerations for critically burned patients. *Crit Care Clin* 1985;**1**(1):3–26.

White CE, Renz EM. Advances in surgical care: management of severe burn injury. *Crit Care Med* 2008;**36**(7 Suppl):S318–24.

INITIAL WOUND CARE
Honari S. Topical therapies and antimicrobials in the management of burn wounds. *Crit Care Nurs Clin North Am* 2004;**16**(1):1–11.

Sheridan RL. Burns and inhalation injury. In: Goldstein B, Edelstein D (eds). Critical Care Considerations in Pediatric Trauma. Supplement to Society of Critical Care Medicine. *Critical Care Med* 2002;**30**(11):S500–514.

ESCHAROTOMIES AND FASCIOTOMIES
Brown RL, Greenhalgh DG, Kagan RJ, Warden GD. The adequacy of limb escharotomies–fasciotomics after referral to a major burn center. *J Trauma* 1994;**37**(6):916–20.

Greenhalgh DG, Warden GD. The importance of intra-abdominal pressure measurements in burned children. *J Trauma* 1994;**36**:685–90.

Orgill DP, Piccolo N. Escharotomy and decompressive therapies in burns. *J Burn Care Res* 2009;**30**(5):759–68.

Sheridan RL, Tompkins RG, McManus WF, Pruitt BA, Jr. Intracompartmental sepsis in burn patients. *J Trauma* 1994;**36**:301–5.

CHAPTER 4
RESUSCITATION PHYSIOLOGY
Benzaquin P. *Holocaust* – the shocking story of the Boston Cocoanut Grove Fire. Henry Holt and Company, NY. 1959, pp. 153–184.

LaLonde C, Nayak U, Hennigan J, Demling R. Antioxidants prevent the cellular deficit produced in response to burn injury. *J Burn Care Rehabil* 1996;**17**:379–83.

Lawrence A, Faraklas I, Watkins H, *et al*. Colloid administration normalizes resuscitation ratio and ameliorates 'fluid creep'. *J Burn Care Res* 2010;**31**(1):40–7.

RESUSCITATION PRACTICE
Alvarado R, Chung KK, Cancio LC, Wolf SE. Burn resuscitation. *Burns* 2009;**35**(1):4–14.

Cohen BJ, Jordan MH, Chapin SD, Cape B, Laureno R. Pontine myelinolysis after correction of hyponatremia during burn resuscitation. *J Burn Care Rehabil* 1991;**12**:153–6.

Greenhalgh DG. Burn resuscitation: the results of the ISBI/ABA survey. *Burns* 2010;**36**(2):176–82.

Huang PP, Stucky FS, Dimick AR, Treat RC, Bessey PQ, Rue LW. Hypertonic sodium resuscitation is associated with renal failure and death. *Ann Surgery* 1995;**221**:543–54; discussion 554–7.

Michell MW, Oliveira HM, Kinsky MP, Vaid SU, Herndon DN, Kramer GC. Enteral resuscitation of burn shock using World Health Organization oral rehydration solution: a potential solution for mass casualty care. *J Burn Care Res* 2006;**27**(6):819–25.

CHAPTER 5
INITIAL EVALUATION OF THE WOUND
Heimbach D, Engrav L, Grube B, Marvin J. Burn depth: a review. *World J Surg* 1992;**16**:10–5.

Monstrey S, Hoeksema H, Verbelen J, Pirayesh A, Blondeel P. Assessment of burn depth and burn wound healing potential. *Burns* 2008;**34**(6):761–9.

Sheridan RL. Evaluating and managing burn wounds. *Dermatol Nurs* 2000;**12**(1):8–21.

Sheridan RL, Petras L, Basha G, *et al*. Planimetry study of the percent of body surface represented by the hand and palm: sizing irregular burns is more accurately done with the palm. *J Burn Care Rehabil* 1995;**16**:605–6.

DETERMINING THE TIME AND NEED FOR OPERATION
Chang KC, Ma H, Liao WC, Lee CK, Lin CY, Chen CC. The optimal time for early burn wound excision to reduce pro-inflammatory cytokine production in a murine burn injury model. *Burns* 2010;**36**(7):1059–66.

Desai MH, Rutan RL, Herndon DN. Conservative treatment of scald burns is superior to early excision. *J Burn Care Rehabil* 1991;**12**:482–4.

Herndon DN, Barrow RE, Rutan RL, Rutan TC, Desai MH, Abston S. A comparison of conservative versus early excision. Therapies in severely burned patients. *Ann Surg* 1989;**209**(5):547–52.

TECHNIQUES OF BURN WOUND EXCISION
Mosier MJ, Gibran NS. Surgical excision of the burn wound. *Clin Plast Surg* 2009;**36**(4):617–25.
Sheridan RL, Szyfelbein SK. Staged high-dose epinephrine clysis is safe and effective in extensive tangential burn excisions in children. *Burns* 1999;**25**:745–8.

TECHNIQUES TO MINIMIZE BLOOD LOSS
Brown RA, Grobbelaar AO, Barker S, Rode H. A formula to calculate blood cross-match requirements for early burn surgery in children. *Burns* 1995;**21**:371–3.
Housinger TA, Lang D, Warden GD. A prospective study of blood loss with excisional therapy in pediatric burn patients. *J Trauma* 1993;**34**:262–3.

GRAFT FIXATION AND POSTOPERATIVE WOUND CARE
Sheridan RL. Comprehensive treatment of burns. *Curr Probl Surg* 2001;**38**(9):657–756.
Sheridan RL, Behringer GE, Ryan CM, *et al*. Effective postoperative protection for grafted posterior surfaces: the quilted dressing. *J Burn Care Rehabil* 1995;**16**:607–9.

SKIN SUBSTITUTES
Boyce ST, Hansbrough JF. Biologic attachment, growth, and differentiation of cultured human epidermal keratinocytes on a graftable collagen and chondroitin-6-sulfate substrate. *Surgery* 1988;**103**:421–31.
Heimbach D, Luterman A, Burke J, *et al*. Artificial dermis for major burns. A multi-center randomized clinical trial. *Ann Surgery* 1988;**208**:313–20.
Herndon DN. Perspectives in the use of allograft. *J Burn Care Rehabil* 1997;**18**:S6–Feb.
Sheridan R. Closure of the excised burn wound: autografts, semipermanent skin substitutes, and permanent skin substitutes. *Clin Plast Surg* 2009,**36**(4):643 51.
Sheridan RL, Choucair RJ. Acellular allograft dermis does not hinder initial engraftment in burn resurfacing and reconstruction. *J Burn Care Rehabil* 1997;**18**:496–9.
Sheridan RL, Heggerty M, Tompkins RG, Burke JF. Artificial skin in massive burns: results at ten years. *Eur J Plast Surg* 1994;**17**:91–3.
Sheridan RL, Morgan JR, Cusik JL, Petras LM, Lydon MM, Tompkins RG. Initial experience with a composite autologous skin subsitute. *Burns* 2001;**27**:421–24.
Sheridan RL, Tompkins RG. Cultured autologous epithelium in patients with burns of ninety percent or more of the body surface. *J Trauma* 1995;**38**:48–50.
Sood R, Roggy D, Zieger M, *et al*. Cultured epithelial autografts for coverage of large burn wounds in eighty-eight patients: the Indiana University experience. *J Burn Care Res* 2010;**31**(4):559–68.

Stiefel D, Schiestl C, Meuli M. Integra Artificial Skin for burn scar revision in adolescents and children. *Burns* 2010;**36**(1):114–20.

CHAPTER 6

INHALATION INJURY
Desai MH, Mlcak RP, Robinson E, *et al*. Does inhalation injury limit exercise endurance in children convalescing from thermal injury? (see comments). *J Burn Care Rehabil* 1993;**14**:12–6.
Parker JC, Hernandez LA, Peevy KJ. Mechanisms of ventilator-induced lung injury. *Crit Care Med* 1993;**21**:131–43.

CARBON MONOXIDE AND CYANIDE EXPOSURES
Barillo DJ, Goode R, Esch V. Cyanide poisoning in victims of fire: analysis of 364 cases and review of the literature. *J Burn Care Rehabil* 1994;**15**:46–57.
Grube BJ, Marvin JA, Heimbach DM. Therapeutic hyperbaric oxygen: help or hindrance in burn patients with carbon monoxide poisoning? *J Burn Care Rehabil* 1988;**9**:249–52.
Scheinkestel CD, Bailey M, Myles PS, *et al*. Hyperbaric or normobaric oxygen for acute carbon monoxide poisoning: a randomised controlled clinical trial (see comments). *Med J Aust* 1999;**170**:203–10.
Sheridan RL, Shank ER. Hyperbaric oxygen treatment: a brief overview of a controversial topic. *J Trauma* 1999;**47**(2):426–435.
Thom SR, Taber RL, Mendiguren II, Clark JM, Hardy KR, Fisher AB. Delayed neuropsychologic sequelae after carbon monoxide poisoning: prevention by treatment with hyperbaric oxygen (see comments). *Ann Emerg Med* 1995;**25**:474–80.

RESPIRATORY FAILURE
Chung K, Renz EM, Cancio LC, Wolf S. Regarding critical care of the burn patient: the first 48 hours. *Crit Care Med* 2010;**38**(4):1225.
Hollingsed TC, Saffle JR, Barton RG, Craft WB, Morris SE. Etiology and consequences of respiratory failure in thermally injured patients. *Am J Surg* 1993;**166**:592–6.
Niederman MS, Torres A, Summer W. Invasive diagnostic testing is not needed routinely to manage suspected ventilator-associated pneumonia. *Am J Respir Crit Care Med* 1994;**150**:565–9.
Palmieri TL. Inhalation injury: research progress and needs. *J Burn Care Res* 2007;**28**(4):549–54.
Sheridan RL, Hurford WE, Kacmarek RM, *et al*. Inhaled nitric oxide in burn patients with respiratory failure. *J Trauma* 1997;**42**:629–34.
Sheridan RL, Kacmarek RM, McEttrick MM, *et al*. Permissive hypercapnia as a ventilatory strategy in burned children: effect on barotrauma, pneumonia, and mortality. *J Trauma* 1995;**39**:854–9.

CHRONIC AIRWAY MANAGMENT
Jones WG, Madden M, Finkelstein J, Yurt RW, Goodwin CW. Tracheostomies in burn patients. *Ann Surg* 1989;**209**:471–4.

Palmieri TL, Jackson W, Greenhalgh DG. Benefits of early tracheostomy in severely burned children. *Crit Care Med* 2002;**30**(4):922–4.

Saffle JR, Morris SE, Edelman L. Early tracheostomy does not improve outcome in burn patients. *J Burn Care Rehabil* 2002;**23**(6):431–8.

Sellers BJ, Davis BL, Larkin PW, Morris SE, Saffle JR. Early prediction of prolonged ventilator dependence in thermally injured patients. *J Trauma* 1997;**43**:899–903.

WEANING AND EXTUBATION

Anene O, Meert KL, Uy H, Simpson P, Sarnaik AP. Dexamethasone for the prevention of postextubation airway obstruction: a prospective, randomized, double-blind, placebo-controlled trial. *Crit Care Med* 1996;**24**:1666–9.

Calhoun KH, Deskin RW, Garza C, *et al*. Long-term airway sequelae in a pediatric burn population. *Laryngoscope* 1988;**98**:721–5.

Sheridan R, Keaney T, Enfanto R. Propofol infusion as an adjunct to extubation in burned children. *J Burn Care Rehabil* 2003;**24**:356–60.

CHAPTER 7

NEUROLOGIC AND PAIN CONTROL ISSUES

Dagum AB, Peters WJ, Neligan PC, Douglas LG. Severe multiple mononeuropathy in patients with major thermal burns. *J Burn Care Rehabil* 1993;**14**:440–5.

Hoffman HG, Patterson DR, Seibel E, Soltani M, Jewett-Leahy L, Sharar SR. Virtual reality pain control during burn wound debridement in the hydrotank. *Clin J Pain* 2008;**24**(4):299–304.

Marquez S, Turley JJ, Peters WJ. Neuropathy in burn patients. *Brain* 1993;**116**:471–83.

Stoddard FM, Martyn JJ, Sheridan RL. Psychiatric issues in pain of burn injury: controlling pain and improving outcomes. *Curr Rev Pain* 1997;**1**:130–6.

Stoddard FJ Jr, Sorrentino EA, Ceranoglu TA, *et al*. Preliminary evidence for the effects of morphine on posttraumatic stress disorder symptoms in one- to four-year-olds with burns. *J Burn Care Res* 2009;**30**(5):836–43.

HEMODYNAMIC AND ELECTROLYTE ISSUES

Burns SM, Fisher C, Earven Tribble SS, *et al*. Multifactor clinical score and outcome of mechanical ventilation weaning trials: burns wean assessment program. *Am J Crit Care* 2010;**19**(5):431–9.

King DR, Namias N, Andrews DM. Coagulation abnormalities following thermal injury. *Blood Coagul Fibrinolysis* 2010;**21**(7):666–9.

Kompoti MG, Michalia MG. Critical care of the burn patient: the first 48 hours. *Crit Care Med* 2010;**38**(5):1391; author reply 1391–2.

Sheridan RL. Critical care of the burn patient. In: Hurford WE, Bigatello LM, Haspel KL, Warren RL (eds). *Critical Care Handbook of the Massachusetts General Hospital*. Philadelphia: Lippincott Williams and Wilkins, 2000, pp. 584–609.

VASCULAR ACCESS ISSUES

Seldinger S. Catheter replacement of the needle in percutaneous arteriography (a new technique). *Acta Radiol* 1953;**39**:368–76.

Sheridan RL, Weber JM. Mechanical and infectious complications of pediatric central venous cannulation: lessons learned from a 10-year experience placing over 1000 central venous catheters in children. *J Burn Care Res* 2006;**27**(5):713–8.

NUTRITIONAL SUPPORT ISSUES

Gilpin DA, Barrow RE, Rutan RL, Broemeling L, Herndon DN. Recombinant human growth hormone accelerates wound healing in children with large cutaneous burns. *Ann Surg* 1994;**220**:19–24.

Greenhalgh DG, Housinger TA, Kagan RJ, *et al*. Maintenance of serum albumin levels in pediatric burn patients: a prospective, randomized trial. *J Trauma* 1995;**39**:67–73.

Pereira CT, Murphy KD, Herndon DN. Altering metabolism. *J Burn Care Rehabil* 2005;**26**(3):194–9.

Prelack K, Dwyer J, Dallal GE, *et al*. Growth decleration and restoration after serious burn injury. *J Burn Care Res* 2007;**28**(2): 262–68.

Prelack K, Dylewski M, Sheridan RL. Practical guidelines for nutritional management of burn injury and recovery. *Burns* 2007;**33**:14–24.

COMPLICATIONS AND SEPSIS

Deitch EA. The role of intestinal barrier failure and bacterial translocation in the development of systemic infection and multiple organ failure. [Review]. *Arch Surg* 1990;**125**:403–4.

Greenhalgh DG, Saffle JR, Holmes JH 4th, *et al*; American Burn Association Consensus Conference on Burn Sepsis and Infection Group. American Burn Association consensus conference to define sepsis and infection in burns. *J Burn Care Res* 2007;**28**(6):776–90.

Sheridan RL, Weber J, Benjamin J, Pasternack MS, Tompkins RG. Control of methicillin-resistant *Staphylococcus aureus* in a pediatric burn unit. *Am J Infection Control* 1994;**22**:340–5.

Weber JM, Sheridan RL, Pasternack MS, Tompkins RG. Nosocomial infections in pediatric patients with burns. *Am J Infection Control* 1997;**25**:195–201.

BURN WOUND INFECTION

Sheridan RL. Sepsis in pediatric burn patients. *Pediatr Crit Care Med* 2005;**6**(3):S112–9.

Sheridan RL, Weber JM, Pasternack MM, Tompkins RG. Antibiotic prophylaxis for group A streptococcal burn wound infection is not necessary. *J Trauma* 2001;**51**:352–5.

CHAPTER 8

FACIAL BURNS

Kung TA, Gosain AK. Pediatric facial burns. *J Craniofac Surg* 2008;**19**(4):951–9.

EYELID BURNS

Achauer BM, Adair SR. Acute and reconstructive management of the burned eyelid. *Clin Plast Surg* 2000;**27**(1):87–96.

Barrow RE, Jeschke MG, Herndon DN. Early release of third-degree eyelid burns prevents eye injury. *Plast Reconstr Surg* 2000;**105**(3):860–3.

EAR BURNS

Skedros DG, Goldfarb IW, Slater H, Rocco J. Chondritis of the burned ear: a review. *Ear Nose Throat J* 1992;**71**(8):359–62.

SCALP BURNS

Pisarski GP, Mertens D, Warden GD, Neale HW. Tissue expander complications in the pediatric burn patient. *Plast Reconstr Surg* 1998;**102**(4):1008–12.

NECK BURNS

Grevious MA, Paulius K, Gottlieb LJ. Burn scar contractures of the pediatric neck. *J Craniofac Surg* 2008;**19**(4):1010–5.

Sheridan RL, Ryan DP, Fuzaylov G, Nimkin K, Martyn JA. Case records of the Massachusetts General Hospital. Case 2-2008. Case 5-2008. An 18-month-old girl with an advanced neck contracture after a burn. *N Engl J Med* 2008;**358**(7):729–35.

HAND BURNS

Sheridan RL, Hurley J, Smith MA, *et al*. The acutely burned hand: management and outcome based on a ten-year experience with 1047 acute hand burns. [Review]. *J Trauma* 1995;**38**:406–11.

GENITAL BURNS

Housinger TA, Keller B, Warden GD. Management of burns of the penis. *J Burn Care Rehabil* 1993;**14**:525–7.

CHAPTER 9

ELECTRICAL INJURIES

Mann R, Gibran N, Engrav L, Heimbach D. Is immediate decompression of high-voltage electrical injuries to the upper extremity always necessary? *J Trauma* 1996;**40**:584–7; discussion 587–9.

Rabban JT, Blair JA, Rosen CL, Adler JN, Sheridan RL. Mechanisms of pediatric electrical injury. New implications for product safety and injury prevention. *Arch Pediatr Adolesc Med* 1997;**151**:696–700.

CHEMICAL BURNS

Mozingo DW, Smith AA, McManus WF, Pruitt BA Jr, Mason AD. Chemical burns. *J Trauma* 1988;**28**(5):642–7.

Sheridan RL, Ryan CM, Quinby WC, Jr., Blair J, Tompkins RG, Burke JF. Emergency management of major hydrofluoric acid exposures. *Burns* 1995;**21**:62–4.

HOT TAR BURNS

Demling RH, Buerstatte WR, Perea A. Management of hot tar burns. *J Trauma* 1980;**20**:242.

Stratta RJ, Saffle JR, Kravitz M, Warden GD. Management of tar and asphalt injuries. *Am J Surg* 1983;**146**:766–9.

COLD INJURIES

Britt LD, Dascombe WH, Rodriguez A. New horizons in the management of hypothermia and frostbite injury. *Surg Clin N Am* 1991;**71**:345–70.

Sheridan RL, Goldstein MA, Stoddard FJ Jr, Walker, Case records of the Massachusetts General Hospital. Case 41-2009. A 16-year-old boy with hypothermia and frostbite. *N Engl J Med* 2009;**361**(27):2654–62.

TOXIC EPIDERMAL NECROLYSIS

Goyal S, Gupta P, Ryan CM, Kazlas M, Noviski N, Sheridan RL. Toxic epidermal necrolysis in children: medical, surgical, and ophthalmologic considerations. *J Burn Care Res* 2009;**30**(3):437–49.

Sheridan RL, Gagnon SW, Tompkins RG. The burn unit as a resource for the management of acute nonburn conditions in children. *J Burn Care Rehabil* 1995;**16**:62–4.

Sheridan RL, Weber JM, Schulz JT, Ryan CM, Low HM, Tompkins RG. Management of severe toxic epidermal necrolysis in children. *J Burn Care Rehabil* 1999;**20**:497–500.

Taylor JA, Grube B, Heimbach DM, Bergman AB. Toxic epidermal necrolysis. A comprehensive approach. Multidisciplinary management in a burn center. *Clin Pediatr* 1989;**28**:404–7.

PURPURA FULMINANS

Aiuto LT, Barone SR, Cohen PS, Boxer RA. Recombinant tissue plasminogen activator restores perfusion in meningococcal purpura fulminans. *Crit Care Med* 1997;**25**:1079–82.

Sheridan RL, Briggs SE, Remensnyder JP, Tompkins RG. Management strategy in purpura fulminans with multiple organ failure in children. *Burns* 1996;**22**:53–6.

STAPHYLOCOCCAL SCALDED SKIN SYNDROME

Sheridan RL, Briggs SE, Remensnyder JP, *et al*. The burn unit as a resource for the management of acute nonburn conditions in children. *J Burn Care Rehabil* 1995;**16**:62–4.

SOFT TISSUE TRAUMA AND INFECTION

Gunter OL, Guillamondegui OD, May AK, Diaz JJ. Outcome of necrotizing skin and soft tissue infections. *Surg Infect* 2008;**9**(4):443–50.

INJURIES OF ABUSE

Hobson MI, Evans J, Stewart IP. An audit of nonaccidental injury in burned children. *Burns* 1994;**20**:442–5.

COMBINED BURNS AND TRAUMA

Rosenkrantz K, Sheridan RL. Management of the burned trauma patient: balancing conflicting priorities. *Burns* 2002;**28**(7):665–9.

CHAPTER 10

PATIENT SELECTION

Coffee T, Yurko L, Fratianne RB. Mixing inpatient with outpatient care: establishing an outpatient clinic on a burn unit. *J Burn Care Rehabil* 1992;**13**:587–9.

Sheridan R. Outpatient burn care in the emergency department. *Pediatr Emerg Care* 2005;**21**(7):449–56.

TECHNIQUES

Waitzman AA, Neligan PC. How to manage burns in primary care. *Can Family Phys* 1993;**39**:2394–400.

CHAPTER 11

EARLY ACUTE REHABILITATION

Esselman PC, Thombs BD, Magyar-Russell G, Fauerbach JA. Burn rehabilitation: state of the science. *Am J Phys Med Rehabil* 2006;**85**(4):383–413.

Salisbury R. Burn rehabilitation: our unanswered challenge. The 1992 presidential address to the American Burn Association. *J Burn Care Rehabil* 1992;**13**:495–505.

LATE ACUTE REHABILITATION

Achauer BM. *Burn Reconstruction*. New York: Thieme Medical Publishers Inc., 1991, pp. 1–188.

Richard RL, Hedman TL, Quick CD, *et al*. A clarion to recommit and reaffirm burn rehabilitation. *J Burn Care Res* 2008;**29**(3):425–32.

LONG TERM REHABILITATION AND SCAR MANAGEMENT

Carr-Collins JA. Pressure techniques for the prevention of hypertrophic scar. *Clin Plast Surg* 1992;**19**:733–43.

Donelan MB, Parrett BM, Sheridan RL. Pulsed dye laser therapy and z-plasty for facial burn scars: the alternative to excision. *Ann Plast Surg* 2008;**60**(5):480–6.

Kischer CW. The microvessels is hypertrophic scars, keloids and related lesions. *J Submicrosc Cytol Path* 1992;**24**:281–96.

McDonald WS, Deitch EA. Hypertrophic skin grafts in burned patients: a prospective analysis of variables. *J Trauma* 1987;**27**:147–50.

Sheridan RL, MacMillan K, Donelan M, *et al*. Tuneable dye laser neovessel ablation as an adjunct to the management of hypertrophic scarring in burned children: pilot trial to establish safety. *J Burn Care Rehabil* 1997;**18**:317–20.

CHAPTER 12

HEAD AND NECK

Achauer BM. Reconstructing the burned face. *Clin Plast Surg* 1992;**19**(3):623–36.

Klein MB, Moore ML, Costa B, Engrav LH. Primer on the management of face burns at the University of Washington. *J Burn Care Rehabil* 2005;**26**(1):2–6.

HAND

Sheridan RL, Baryza MJ, Pessina MA, *et al*. Acute hand burns in children: management and long-term outcome based on a 10-year experience with 698 injured hands. *Ann Surg* 1999;**229**:558–64.

UPPER EXTREMITY

Hunt JL, Arnoldo BD, Kowalske K, Helm P, Purdue GF. Heterotopic ossification revisited: a 21-year surgical experience. *J Burn Care Res* 2006;**27**(4):535–40.

Lindenhovius AL, Linzel DS, Doornberg JN, Ring DC, Jupiter JB. Comparison of elbow contracture release in elbows with and without heterotopic ossification restricting motion. *J Shoulder Elbow Surg* 2007;**16**(5):621–5.

LOWER EXTREMITY

Peterson SL, Mani MM, Crawford CM, Neff JR, Hiebert JM. Postburn heterotopic ossification: insights for management decision making. *J Trauma* 1989;**29**:365–9.

AFTERCARE AND EMOTIONAL RECOVERY

Baker CP, Rosenberg M, Mossberg KA, *et al*. Relationships between the Quality of Life Questionnaire (QLQ) and the SF-36 among young adults burned as children. *Burns* 2008;**34**(8):1163–8.

Blakeney PE, Rosenberg L, Rosenberg M, Faber AW. Psychosocial care of persons with severe burns. *Burns* 2008;**34**(4):433–40.

Esselman PC, Askay SW, Carrougher GJ, *et al*. Barriers to return to work after burn injuries. *Arch Phys Med Rehabil* 2007;**88**(12 Suppl 2):S50–6.

Fauerbach JA, Lezotte D, Hills RA, *et al*. Burden of burn: a norm-based inquiry into the influence of burn size and distress on recovery of physical and psychosocial function. *J Burn Care Rehabil* 2005;**26**(1):21–32.

Rizzone LP, Stoddard FJ, Murphy JM, Kruger LJ. Post-traumatic stress disorder in mothers of children and adolescents with burns. *J Burn Care Rehabil* 1994;**15**:158–63.

Stoddard FJ, Stroud L, Murphy JM. Depression in children after recovery from severe burns. *J Burn Care Rehabil* 1992;**13**:340–7.

ABBREVIATIONS

BMR basal metabolic rate
CT computed tomography
D5RL 5% dextrose in Ringer's lactate
ECG electrocardiogram
FAST focused assessment with sonography for trauma
HEENT head, eyes, ears, nose, throat
ICU intensive care unit
IP interphalangeal
MCP metacarpophalangeal

MTP metatarsophalangeal
NSAID nonsteroidal anti-inflammatory drug
PEEP positive end-expiratory pressure
RASS Richmond Agitation Sedation Scale
RL Ringer's lactate
SSS staphylococcal scalded skin syndrome
TBSA total body surface area
TEN toxic epidermal necrolysis
WHO World Health Organization

INDEX